Living My Best Life

A Collection of Reader-Submitted Medical Stories

Kerry Hamm

<u>Warning:</u>

This edition features light profanity that may be offensive to some readers. The profanity has been used sparingly and in each instance the usage was included in the submission. I have chosen to leave some of these words in to emphasize portions of the stories.

By now, I am sure you are all too familiar with my *Real Stories from a Small-Town ER* series, which were collections of stories told to you from my time as a registration clerk in Ohio. If you are new here, don't fret! You don't have to worry about a 'certain order' for *any* of my books, including this one!

I have since moved on from the hospital scene, but that hasn't stopped readers from submitting stories of their own experiences from the medical field. Over time, I have received hundreds of stories-some funny, some sad, some downright scary or grotesque-and have worked with my readers to bring these stories to you in a follow up to my last *Real Stories* volume.

If I've learned anything from writing my series and compiling this book, it's that none of us are alone. We're all proof that we've seen some seriously messed up things out there, right? We have seen the good. We've seen the bad. We've seen the downright vile and disgusting. And then, we've seen the humor in these situations and we've been fortunate enough to share them with one another. There is a certain peace in knowing that as no matter how crazy we feel, we have formed solidarity amongst ourselves, knowing that for every bad day you've had, others have had them too. We have worked through the challenges of getting up and facing another drug seeker, another child abuse case, another young death, and another 'how the heck did that even happen?' moment together. You guys are not alone, and this book reaffirms that.

Several of the stories have been edited to bring you clear-cut and clean versions of tales submitted by loyal readers. I have done my very best to edit out hospital and town names, and in some cases my submitters wished to withhold their initials and other details from publication or requested that I edit stories for grammar/spelling. Some stories have been edited for length. I do my very best to preserve a reader's humor and emotions, as well as capture the reader's personality when I edit these submissions. To be clear, I do my best to remove ANY identifying information from these submissions, and sometimes that may include altering specific stand-out details with the submitter's permission. This is to prevent readers from searching for patients online, thus revealing the identities of parties involved. This is done carefully, and I work with readers to keep touchy submissions as close to the initial submission as possible.

Though some of the stories in this collection are horrifying, I am glad none of us are alone in what we've witnessed or experienced.

<u>**Cheat Sheet**</u>

Some readers have been confused about terms used in this series. Here's a quick list to help you out!

LEO: Law Enforcement Officer

ETOH: shorthand for Ethyl Alcohol or Ethanol; commonly used to describe intoxicated individuals

Bus/Rig/Truck: Ambulance

M.D.: Medical Doctor

R.N.: Registered Nurse

MVA: Motor Vehicle Accident

EMS: Emergency Medical Services

EMT: Emergency Medical Technician

PD/FD: Police Department/Fire Department

D.A.: District Attorney

BOLO: Be on (the) Lookout

DCFS/CPS: Department of Children and Family Services/Child Protective Services

SNF: Skilled Nursing Facility. This can be a nursing home or one of many facilities for patients in need of supervised care

AMA: Against Medical Advice

LWBS/LBT: Left Without Being Seen/Left Before Triage

LOL: Little Old Lady

<u>Pudding Cups</u>

I was returning a cart to the supply closet at the SNF where I work, when I came up on a room and heard two of my residents bickering.

From what I could gather, Jane (who suffered from dementia) was accusing Joan of stealing and eating her pudding cup from her tray as the two ate lunch and watched television from their beds.

"I didn't eat your pudding," Joan snapped. "*You* ate your pudding, you forgetful, miserable cow."

I was fully prepared to enter the room to play mediator, but Jane thought for a second before laughing and replied, "You know, I think you might be right!"

-O.R.

Wisconsin

<u>Not Stressed</u>

I was drawing blood on a guy one morning and noticed he was straining. He made audible grunting, was clenching his teeth, and his eyes looked like they were going to pop out of his head.

Because of his age (he was in his late-40s to early-50s), I couldn't imagine that this was his first draw. So, I smiled and asked, "Do blood draws make you uneasy?"

He looked confused and said, "No. Why?"

I mentioned that I noticed he was straining and looked uncomfortable.

With a straight face, he told me, "My butthole itches, so I'm trying to fart."

I was so unprepared for his explanation that I stopped paying attention to what I was doing and ended up with blood all over my gloves and his arm. I scrambled to get us both

cleaned up and apologized. He didn't seem
fazed at all.

-T.P.-K.

Oklahoma

<u>The Text Message</u>

I've been with the PD for 22 years, and I've seen it all. I've heard it all. *C.O.P.S* has nothin' on what we've seen on our runs. I thought I'd share one of the lighter moments I've experienced during my time with the station.

An elderly man entered the station one day, and since I wasn't busy, I offered to assist him with his needs.

When I asked what brought him in that morning, he said with a sigh, "Someone's stalking my wife."

"Stalking your wife?" I asked.

He nodded and pointed to an elderly woman who was seated in a chair at the front of the station.

"He keeps texting my wife," the man explained. "She reads it, but she doesn't reply."

"What do the texts say?" I asked.

4

"Same thing, over and over," he said. "Just says, "Hi! Do you want to meet for lunch?" She never responds. You'd think he'd take the hint by now, right?"

I nodded and asked, "Is it someone you or your wife know?"

The man shook his head hard and said, "No. No. We've both been over this a billion times. We've been through both our address books. We don't know nobody named Jonathan."

"Okay," I said. "Have you thought of maybe replying, just to tell him he has the wrong number? When your wife got her phone, maybe she got a phone number that used to belong to Jonathan's friend or something."

"Haven't tried that," the man said. "We don't want to talk to him."

The old man motioned for his wife. She shuffled over and reached in her handbag. She handed me the biggest cell phone I'd ever seen. It was built like an old Nokia. It felt like I was holding an old graphing calculator. It was clear the phone was one of those 'special' phones for elderly users. It didn't seem to have internet capability (from what I could tell), and it didn't have a speaker or camera from what I could see.

"See," the old man said, tapping on the screen, "He sent the damned text again! My Jane is a married gal. She's taken. Not about to lose her over a Reuben."

Jane nodded and said with a chuckle, "That's right. We've been married for 72 years. I'm too old to be chasing another man. Besides, I've kind of grown fond of this one."

I hit a few buttons on the cell phone and noticed that no matter which button I pressed, the message on the screen stayed the same.

It took me about five more seconds to realize why.

Using my nails, I carefully peeled off a protective screen cover that was pre-printed with the message, "Hi! Do you want to meet for lunch? Jonathan."

The phone's owner had three unread text messages from her family, and she had a few missed calls. The couple asked me to help them set up their voice mailbox, so I helped

them program that before they thanked me for
my time and went on their merry way.

-C.S.
California

<u>Secret Agent Man</u>

On my first night as ED Registrar, about an hour or two into the shift, I had a man come to the desk and demand a prescription for narcotics. I could tell he was pretty messed up on drugs or something, so I tried to call security. The man realized that I was reaching for the phone, and he reached over the desk and yanked the entire phone from my desk. He threw it on the floor.

I had worked night audit at hotels for years, so I was used to dealing with weird people. I was not, however, used to dealing with violent people, and I had virtually no training. I was literally interviewed the day before, drug tested and hired that morning, and then I was scheduled for my first shift alone that night. I was scared out of my mind and had no idea what to do.

There was a door not far away, but I didn't know if my badge would work to open it because I already knew I had trouble accessing other rooms, like the supply closet and a door that would let me go to another hall to use the bathroom.

At this point, all I could do was pray that someone else came inside, that security arrived, or that someone from the treatment area saw the man's actions on their cameras.

The man started speaking in gibberish. The only coherent thing I could understand him saying was, "I'm a freaking ninja! You don't know who you're messing with!"

He started hopping around and was trying to do karate kicks in the lobby. He then ran to the lobby entrance, and I started thinking he was going to leave. He did not.

Instead, he started running towards my desk, tried to do a flip, and he hit his head on the corner of my desk. My desk moved about three inches (which surprised me; I thought it was stationary), and the man was out cold on the floor. He was bleeding from a wound to the head, but it wasn't as bad as you'd think it would be. There really wasn't much blood.

I tried to enter the treatment area, but the badge reader flashed red. I felt trapped because at that time of night, the *only* way in or out of the hospital is through the ED lobby entrance area. My phone was smashed to pieces on the lobby floor, and nobody seemed to hear me as I banged on the doors to the treatment area.

I saw a cell phone next to the man's body, so I did the only thing I could think to do, and I used his phone to call 911. I explained the situation and said that since it was after midnight, I couldn't walk around the hospital to find another phone.

The 911 operator called the hospital's main line and asked the operator to get security and help to my area. She said she was sending the police, too.

I guess the patient told the doctor that he'd recently taken LSD and cocaine.

I thought most of the nurses would be nice to me following the incident, but it became somewhat of a bullying situation and they were incredibly rude. One nurse said I was dumb, and another one asked, "Why didn't you just call us on the waiting room phone?" She rolled her eyes and walked away after I told her that nobody had even told me there was a phone in the waiting room.

My boss yelled at me for 1.) touching the patient's personal property, and 2.) allowing him to break hospital property. She tried to tell me that she was going to dock my pay for the cost of the phone because she didn't think it was fair to make the department pay for *my* error. I told the lady that it was suddenly clear why I'd been hired so quickly, and I told her I quit. I left her office and immediately filed a complaint with H.R. They were so concerned with my account of the events (that the police, switchboard operator, and one anonymous nurse from the treatment area confirmed) that they offered me a job in their department.

Everything worked in my favor. I finally got a day job, was paid more for the new position, and I didn't have to put up with that craziness anymore.

-Initials and location withheld at request

<u>Saline Drip</u>

This is my story about the saline drip. Now I know these saline drips comes in all sorts of recipes and flavors, with different names from all sorts of suppliers and manufacturers, but for a non-medic like myself, I'll just call it saline drip.

We live in a normal sized town of about thirty thousand inhabitants and I work as an electrician. My father-in-law was one of the family doctors from the area. His daughter, my wife, was a radiologist. We all lived together in the same large house. About once every eight weeks my father-in-law had emergency standby duty.

As he was getting on a bit, I used to ride shotgun with him on calls when I was available. Those days you fixed your broken fingernails yourself and emergencies were emergencies. The EMTs were always on scene first and my dad-in-law had to make legal decisions. Very often I was left holding a bag of saline drip in the air. I never knew what for.

My wife and I bought a large old timber framed house that was a stone's throw away from the volunteer fire department. Pretty soon I was roped in.

Our firehouse building is seven truck bays wide and fronted by a 100 ft deep practice area that separates us from a feeder road to a freeway intersection.

Not much catches fire these days and most calls are MVAs on the local freeway. If I was in my study when the pager went off, I would bound down the stairs two at a time and sprint to the firehouse and try and get a driver's seat.

I was quick, however there were many times others were quicker and I saw taillights with flashing toplights leaving the bay. I then manned the next fire truck. A few of these times I ended up being the guy holding the saline drip.

Among all the volunteer fire folks we have here are all sorts of various professions.

Although we do not run any medical trucks from our station, we do however have about half a dozen professional EMTs in our ranks.

This, I suspect, is because I think they get accredited hours for turning up on exercise nights as well as the fact that the beer is cheap after training. Sometimes the beer is actually free if we get a crate donated from the appreciative community or from one of our grateful customers.

Do not get the impression we would ever drink and drive.

Like myself, a lot of us live within a walking, or maybe sometimes a sprinting, distance of the fire station.

A further sobering aspect is that the police regularly use our floodlight parking lot around the back as a temporary car pound for their, maybe not so grateful, customers.

The police use our large practice area at the front as a pull off staging area checking cars coming from the freeway heading home.

It was during these beer sessions that the EMTs would talk about what they did and why, but I still had the impression that whatever else, their customers ended up with a cervical collar and a saline drip.

One late sunny Saturday afternoon I was doing my post when I opened a nasty letter from the tax authorities. Nothing special but worrying. I waved their paper out of the window at my wife Jane who was clearing the yard below.

I bounded down the stairs four at a time instead of my usual two at a time when the fire department pager goes off. The last five steps however were taken with a leap toward the open door to the yard where my wife was waiting for me.

I smashed my head into a wooden beam about the size and shape of a large roof gutter. No blood. No pain. Just "thud".

I knew this bump was now going to swell up. My wife got an ice pack.

While rolling this flat blue square plastic block of frozen water around my skull I realised it was not working liked we hoped for.

With visualisations of my head opening up like Vesuvius spurting blood on all sides, I went down to the cellar and rummaged around in the freezer. There I found this old squashed 2-liter Coke bottle.

The bottle had a label on it that read "Ouzo". The freezer was about 0F which is about -18C.

This Coke bottle was so formed that it had the shape of a matador hat. You know the caps the toreros wear at the bull fights. A perfect fit.

We hit the road and I felt OK for the first mile. It was when I tried to check the fit of my new headgear that I realised it was frozen to my summer crew cut. Not wanting to get to the ER like an idiot, it dawned on me that the EMTs have a staging outpost behind the freeway services.

It is just a container with a car port with outside power sockets for an ambulance. Because it can be reached via the delivery backroads, you can get from there to almost anywhere very quickly.

We rolled up.

A large lady in white stood up.

"Is John here?" I asked.

"I don't know a John" She replied.

"Do you know Jim?" Was my next question.

"We're from a station from the other side of town. What's up?"

I proceeded to explain that I had bust my head open and now had a Coke bottle frozen to my skull.

The lady in white first peered at me then slid the side door of her ambulance open, she reached in and pulled out…, you've guessed it, a saline drip.

I stared in horror at this shiny bag raised above her head glistening against the late afternoon sun. A tube jingle jangled around her knees.

"No, no I ain't that far gone." I stuttered as I tried to protect my blood donor veins by clasping over my elbows with my hands. My wife had disappeared as I looked at this apparition in panic.

"Sir. We don't have any hot water here." She said. "This stuff is blood temperature. Bend over please."

17

I felt my wife gently pushing me towards the nurse.

"No needles." I begged.

"Bend over." she repeated commandingly.

The ride to ER was uneventful. The swelling had subsided, and I got a 6cm starburst glued up.

I signed out saying it was our decision to leave without X-ray.

Now getting on a bit myself, whenever I see that wound through my thinning grey hair, it is with a fond smile that I remember that saline drip.

-D.E.
Location withheld

Go to Sleep (Or I Will Put You to Sleep)

Only a few of us were at the station, and we were playing a game of non-alcoholic beer pong with grape soda and orange juice that we'd found in the fridge. The phone rang, and I didn't want to have to chug another Dixie cup of generic pop, so I ran clear across the station in about 1.4 seconds to answer the call.

"County EMS," I answered.

The caller sounded like she was in her thirties. I couldn't quite make out everything at first because there was so much screaming going on in the background.

"You're gonna be sorry when I'm done on this phone!" she yelled.

"Hello?" I asked.

With an attitude she snapped, "You could at least give me a second to talk, you know."

"How can I help you?" I asked.

"I need some ketamine," she told me.

I laughed and said, "Ma'am, did you know that you called EMS?"

She went off on a profanity-laced tirade and said she knew exactly who she'd called.

"I have three kids under eight," she said to me. "I've been telling them to go to bed for two hours, but they want to be stuck-up little bastards about it, and they won't sleep."

"Okay…," I said. "I'm not sure I can help you with that, ma'am."

She snapped again and told me, "Yes, you can. I just told you that I needed ketamine. I know you have it. I'm not stupid."

"Ma'am," I said, clearly agitated, "I cannot bring ketamine to your house because you can't get your kids to go to sleep."

My partner and coworkers stopped what they were doing to just stare at me.

The woman on the line cursed some more, and right before I was about to hang up on her, she screamed to me, "Fine. If you can't do this one simple [effing] thing for me, then maybe I'll just beat them until you have to come and take them to the hospital. Maybe I'll start with my two-year-old and drown him in the tub. Hope you feel good about that when you read it in the news tomorrow!"

I told the woman we could bring her drugs 'just one time,' and she became a totally different person.

As soon as I got her address and name, I hung up and called the police department to report the caller and the threats she made against her children.

Nobody from EMS visited the home, but two police officers did, and they called in CPS because the children showed evidence of abuse. The officers also arrested the caller that night because she had drugs laid out on the coffee table when she invited the officers inside.

From what I understand, the kids were initially separated and placed with foster families, but one of the families petitioned the courts and asked that the children be fostered together for their wellbeing. I think the caller is still in jail because she had felony warrants out for her.

That's honestly the craziest thing I've ever experienced in EMS, aside from the addicts we get every now and then.

-T.J.

Tennessee

<u>We Don't Say That Here</u>

I transferred to a rural town after having spent my entire life hopping from big city to big city.   I suspected it wasn't the life for me on my first day of work at my new EMS station.

"My husband's Nigerian," I told one of my coworkers, as I was explaining our holiday plans.

Everyone in the room stopped talking. Finally, one young girl leaned in with a disgusted look on her face and said, "Look, I know you were probably around a lot of different kinds of people where you used to work, and I know your husband probably doesn't mind, but that doesn't mean that you can say that word."

Someone filed a complaint with my new boss, and I had to pull up a map on my phone to show my boss that the Federal Republic of

Nigeria is a (real) *place,* and I **was not** using a racial slur.

When I went home and told my husband about it, he started laughing because he thought I'd made up the story as a joke. He didn't believe me until I showed him a copy of my 'counseling report' that I'd received from my boss.

We didn't stay long, but it didn't have much to do with my job. My husband and I simply couldn't get used to small-town life.

-P.Z.

California

<u>Go Team!</u>

My partner and I staged at a college sporting event on Christmas Eve. The team won, and everyone was celebrating in the locker room. We decided to grab a few autographs before we left.

All the sudden, the room erupted with, "Chug! Chug! Chug!"

When I turned around, I saw one of the guys from the team chugging whisky straight from the bottle.

"You should probably not do that," I said. My words were lost in the crowd.

It had been a full bottle of hard liquor, and the guy had it all gone in about 30 seconds.

My partner sighed and said, "We should probably stick around because you know this isn't gonna be good."

He was right, of course. Twenty minutes later, we had the guy loaded up in the back of the ambulance. He was covered in vomit, and I had to hold an emesis bag to his face so that I wouldn't have to clean out our vehicle. The ER kept him for observation. I don't know if he was even supposed to have alcohol in the locker room, so I've been wondering if he'll get in trouble for that.

Oh well, at least I got to attend a free game and had floor seats.

-R.F.

Indiana

Deck the Halls

Dispatch sent me across town to a domestic complaint, and as soon as I stepped foot in the residence, I called for EMS transport and additional officers.

There was a full-out brawl taking place in this two-bedroom apartment. The Christmas tree had been knocked over during the brawl, and it had busted out one of the windows. There were broken ornaments all over the floor, as well as spilled drinks, food, and blood.

I tried to create order in the residence, but four college-aged females were going at it, and it was a bloodbath. Hair had been torn out in patches, one girl was missing teeth, all four looked like they'd been beaten to hell, and two of the females had bites to their arms and legs from a medium-sized dog that had given up on the fight and was standing guard between the kitchen and living room.

When additional officers arrived, we managed to get the ladies pulled apart. It wasn't easy. In fact, we had to deploy tasers on two of the women (one became combative with officers, and one tried to run).

We got everyone zip-tied and lined up on the couch while we awaited EMS. At this point, the extent of the wounds was more visible, and it was bad. One of the females had bitten another's lip and yanked a lip piercing right out of her face, leaving the lady's face torn and bleeding profusely.

None of the women seemed to understand how to shut up. Despite being restrained and knowing they were going to jail, they continued bickering and the two who'd not been tased continued to fight by headbutting and kicking one another. We had to separate the women further by moving them to opposite sides of the room.

You wouldn't believe what started this fight.

Wrapping paper.

That's right. Wrapping paper.

One of the women had received a gift wrapped in festive red paper that had, "Ho, Ho, Ho!" written on it in bold white lettering.

From what I could gather, she received that gift from her roommate who "did that shit on purpose" after the roommate found out the woman had sex with her longtime crush.

Come to find out, if it hadn't been the wrapping paper that started the brawl, I'm absolutely positive it would have been the gift.

The roommate had somehow gained access to the woman's Cloud storage service and had printed out hundreds of photos that were sexual in nature, had a bunch of screenshots of texts printed out, and I guess she included pictures of envelopes that she'd taken before she sent copies of the photos and screenshots to the woman's parents, ex-boyfriend, current boyfriend, and some of the woman's college professors. Some of the women were in more trouble than others, obviously.

A nosy neighbor came over, and surprisingly, all four girls agreed to allow the neighbor to care for the 'house dog' until one of them could be bailed out.

EMS transported three of the females to the ER, and we transported the fourth. All four received medical attention. All four needed sutures, and that was just a base starting point for treatment.

Three of the women were released from the hospital and then transported to jail. One of the women was kept for observation, following complications from being tased. We were called back to the hospital just a short time later because she had tried to leave the hospital wearing nothing but her gown (they took her clothes so she wouldn't try to leave, but you see how well that worked), and then she punched a tech who'd tried to stop her from leaving.

I would like to stress that I was only working this shift because one of my coworkers wanted to spend time with his pregnant wife. If I hadn't been such a nice guy and offered to pick up his shift, I would have been in bed while these women were going MMA on each other. I think he owes me big time. I'll gladly accept Starbucks gift cards, Greg.

-I.G.

Location withheld at request

Fur Baby

We all joke about it, but our patient's wife did it.

When we told her she could not bring the family dog in to visit her husband, she became upset and left.

An hour later, she returned with this 20-pound dog dressed in a snowsuit. She was pushing him in a stroller, and he was covered with a blanket.

"Ma'am," I said, "you can't take your dog on the floor."

She looked me dead in the eyes and said, "Dog? This is my grandson, thank you very much."

'Really? Because his ears, fur, and whiskers say otherwise,' I thought.

The lady's husband had only been admitted for four hours, anyway, so her stunt was more annoying than anything else.

Her husband was discharged the next day, and they both wrote us scathing reviews online, as well as left all one-stars on the patient satisfaction report.

-T.R.

Ohio

The other day, my partner and I were dispatched to a mental health call.

As we approached the address, we witnessed someone dressed in one of those inflatable dinosaur costumes running down the sidewalk, chasing a potbellied pig that was on a harness and leash.

"This must be it," I said, pulling over.

A lady across the street waved her arms and shouted, "Over here!"

We were at the wrong house.

-Y.E.

Illinois

New Mom Probs

I was supposed to be conducting a six-week exam on a newborn. When I walked in the exam room, it was painfully obvious that the patient's mother was not handling the task of new motherhood very well.

Mom's eyes were red and swollen. She was fidgeting, and she must have sighed and apologized about 30 times in a minute. She used her foot to rock a blanket-covered car seat that she'd placed on the floor.

"Tell me about your health first," I said to the mother.

Her phone rang, and she began sobbing. I could hardly understand her at times, but the gist of it was she was tired, sore, overwhelmed, and on top of it all, she was scared that she was failing as a new mom. She said her marriage was strained because her husband was working all the time and couldn't contribute around the house as much as he wanted, and it was clear that this mother was suffering from postpartum depression. Her phone rang again, and she cried harder.

"We got in a fight before I left," she told me. "And now he won't stop calling me."

She explained that she and her husband were very much in love and that he'd always been very kind to her, but she wanted to be left alone. At the same time, she explained, she didn't want to be left alone. Mom cried so hard that she vomited into a trash can. Throughout the breakdown and the vomiting, she never once stopped rocking the car seat with her foot. When her phone rang again, she turned it off.

We took about 30 minutes to discuss medication options, and we also discussed ways to reduce stress and battle the feelings of isolation, stress, and fear that she was facing.

Once the mother calmed down and seemed accepting of our treatment plan for herself, I said to her, "Okay, get that baby up on the table."

Mom removed the blanket from the car seat and started sobbing all over again. Something in me thought the worst, and every muscle in my body froze at the thought that the baby had stopped breathing or something of the sort. I've been in practice for 37 years and have never been more afraid in my life.

It took about 10 seconds for that fear to subside and for the physician in me to kick in. I looked down, fully preparing myself to snatch a blue-skinned infant from the car seat...only to see that the car seat was empty.

That's right, Kerry. Mom was so stressed out that she'd forgotten to bring the baby to its checkup. While fighting with her husband, she'd managed to remember to grab the car seat, blanket, diaper bag, breast pump, car keys, and her purse...but she forgot to bring the baby.

Her husband had been calling her repeatedly to tell her that the baby was still asleep in the bassinet.

Once this mother realized her blunder, it was sob-city for an hour, and I say that without exaggeration. There was nothing I nor any of my staff could do or say to calm this woman. We simply had to wait it out.

My staff and I shared our own stories about 'parenting fails,' and that seemed to help the mother relax a little. We assured her that we weren't judging her ability to parent, nor did the situation at hand make her a bad mother.

I'm happy to conclude by sharing that this mother accepted treatment for depression and was able to ask for help from her family members. Mom and baby were doing well during the last appointment, and I have no reason to believe that will change.

-K.N., M.D.

Montana

"You can't put me in jail. I'm an influencer [on the internet]."

Sweetie, maybe you should influence people not to do lines of cocaine while they're driving.

-Initials and location withheld at request

The Package

I live in a quiet neighborhood where there are rarely any problems, but as holidays approach, we have an issue with packages being stolen off porches. Because I work the overnight shift, I'm unable to meet package delivery workers when they drop off my packages. Unfortunately, this year has been the worst in the five years I've lived here. I had six packages stolen off my porch in a month. Luckily, most retailers and/or package delivery services worked with me to either refund my money or send replacements. Some did not, and I was out about $200 because someone stole an electronic gift that the FedEx man hid behind a potted plant. I was mad, to say the least.

I was venting about this problem while I was at work, and the House Supervisor heard me. She suggested that I have my packages mailed to my work and assured me that if anyone had a problem with it, she would tell them she gave me permission.

I ordered something and received a text from a coworker on days to let me know she placed the package on our desk with a sticky note that had my name on it. That worked perfectly because I was scheduled to work that night. I told her I'd grab the package while I was at work, thanked her, and I went back to bed.

My job is basically 'overflow' tasks. Because our hospital works with a skeleton crew on nights, I am the hospital switchboard operator, ED registration, a visitor escort, borderline security, and a tech. I don't love my job, but I don't hate it.

I had just returned to my desk from cleaning an ED room, only to see a man had swiped my package from my desk. He saw that I saw him, and he took off running down the corridor. Man, I was hot!

I knew I couldn't chase him down, so I experienced what my supervisor put in the report as a 'temporary lack of judgment' and used the loud speaker microphone to call him out.

This is where I should explain that I've been single for a year. I'm also very confident with myself and with my sexuality. However, I've never been much of a 'single play' kind of person, so when I'm single, I abstain from sexual pleasure. The dry spell was getting the best of me, so I finally gave in and ordered something to solve my problem until I could meet someone new.

I called over the loudspeaker, "Hey asshole, you just stole my vibrator. Bring it back."

As soon as I said the words, I realized that I had just addressed the entire hospital— sleeping patients, staff, everyone—at 03:30. Everyone in the hospital knew I was the only switchboard operator on nights that week, and now they knew that I had a sex toy delivered to me at work.

H.R. said 'no fewer than three' hospital employees filed complaints regarding my foul language, and that one patient threatened to sue the hospital because she had been 'shocked to hear' what I had to say and said that she started having chest pains. I don't doubt the part about the hospital employees, but nobody from the floor where the supposed patient was admitted seemed to know anything about it, so I think they were just trying to make me feel worse about something I was already somewhat embarrassed about. Don't get me wrong, I don't care that people know what I ordered, and I don't care that they know that I had it delivered to work. I was just embarrassed that I had made a hospital-wide announcement in the middle of the night.

So, as an early Christmas gift, I received a write-up. I really didn't get in much trouble. I think most of that was because my supervisor wrote in her report that I do a good job and never cause any problems.

Oh, right after I said that over the loud speaker, the man looked disgusted, and he threw my package on the ground before he ran outside. I didn't get a great look at him, so it's possible that I've encountered him since then.

I'm still allowed to have packages delivered to my job, but my supervisor told me that maybe in the future we should designate a secure location for their safekeeping.

-Initials and location withheld at request

Today, a frequent flyer demanded to be seen ahead of the 20 people in front of him. He said that he visited us so often that he should be on our 'preferred customers' list, and he wanted perks to include no waiting, free socks, and free snacks.

This isn't an amusement park, dude. You don't just get to skip to the front of the line because you come in here every 26 hours for something ridiculous.

-C.B.

Florida

L&D

Two years ago, I was beyond stressed about making a transition from ER RN to L&D. I'd been in ER for four years and when it was good, it was great. Most of my coworkers were awesome, the job was rewarding, I met my fiancée (an EMT) there, and yeah, the carry-ins were nice.

When it was bad, though, it was *bad*. Sometimes people just die, and there's nothing you or anyone else could have done to save them. Sometimes, even six minutes of chest compressions won't save someone. Sometimes, performing emergency CPR on a two-year-old on the ER lobby floor after she'd been pulled out of the pool by her babysitter doesn't work. Coworkers can be nasty to one another, judgmental, hateful. A lot of RNs in this hospital come with a superiority complex. Working 20 to 21 days on and 10 off takes a toll on the body. Being followed to my car was never fun. It also wasn't fun when I had to sign in as a patient because my drug-seeker patient punched me in the face and cracked one of my teeth. It hurt to see Mr. Smith, the local homeless patient, in for the 10th time in three days because it was snowing outside, and he couldn't get help from outreach programs. It wasn't fun to have to turn him away and explain that it was because medically, there wasn't a reason to keep him.

I decided to take the plunge and go to L&D. I was scared, and I quickly learned that I had a reason to be. L&D is hard work.

I soon learned that I wasn't very good at comforting a patient in labor. I learned that I didn't know how to handle being in the room as a mother delivered her stillborn child. I wasn't at all prepared for a mother to scream, "Just take it away!" because she was giving her baby up for adoption.

It took some time to become comfortable on the floor. My coworkers have been excellent from day one. Everyone was/is supportive, and they gave me advice to not only help myself get through tough times, but also to help patients. I hesitate to tell you that it became 'easier' to deal with everything I just mentioned, but in a way, it was 'easier.' I learned how to replace negative emotions and negative energy by delivering positive vibes to my patients.

After a few months, I was 100% positive that I had made the right choice to transition.

A few days ago, something happened.

A family came to the floor, where mom was delivering her fifth baby, a girl after four boys. You'd think by the time you have that many kids that you'd be ready to just go with the flow, but dad was a mess. He was panicky, nervous, sweaty…The man wasn't taking this very well. Our patient, who was in active labor and was halfway there to push, was spending time between contractions yelling at three of her children. The fourth child, who was about four-years-old, sat in the corner with a scowl and crossed his arms.

Grandma and grandpa showed up and took the kids to the waiting room. I was all over the floor that day and had finally gotten a few minutes to sit down and eat lunch. Wouldn't you know, as soon as I sat down, there was that four-year-old standing at my work station, just staring at me.

Finally, I asked, "Do you need help, buddy?"

He nodded and leaned in. With a whisper, he said, "I need to tell you a secret."

I was thinking the worst. I didn't know if this kid was going to tell me he'd pooped his pants or possibly tell me that someone touched him inappropriately. Maybe he was going to pull one of my nephew's moves and his secret was going to be, "I'm hungry. I like chicken wings. Can I have one?"

I leaned in, so the child could tell me his 'secret.'

He reached in his pocket and pulled out a plastic sandwich bag that was filled with pennies, Hot Wheels cars, and yellow Starburst candies. He handed me the bag and said, "This is all I have. Can you send my new sister back?"

Tears filled his eyes and he said, "But you can't tell my mommy, or she will be sad."

The boy's grandma saw that he was 'pestering' me (her words, not mine), and she came over to ask what he was doing and to tell him to let me do my work. This kid had a full-blown meltdown, and it was all because he didn't want his mother to deliver a 'girl baby.'

Grandpa went on a walk around the hospital with the boy, and when they came back, the child seemed to be in a better mood. That all changed when the parents announced the birth of their 6-pound, 8-ounce daughter. The boy cried when he met his sister, and he refused to hold her.

As I was leaving my shift for the day, I heard the boy ask his grandmother, "But can't the doctor give her a pee-pee so she can be a boy?"

I was tickled to death by this little boy and wanted to share the story with everyone. It's really moments like this that make my job fun, exciting, and worthwhile. For all the bad that happens in the world, it sure is worth it to be able to help bring new life into the world. I don't regret transitioning to this department. In fact, I wish I would have done it sooner.

-F.C.

Illinois

Flowery Fight

I responded to an unusual domestic today. A boyfriend and girlfriend were arguing so loudly that their neighbor called 911.

When I arrived, the boyfriend explained that he and his girlfriend had attended a wedding. The two were arguing over catching the bride's bouquet.

You're probably thinking that the girlfriend caught the bouquet and was now insisting the two get married. Wrong.

The girlfriend did not participate in the bouquet throw, and her boyfriend was upset because, "It's like you tried to tell everyone there that you don't want to marry me."

She screamed (almost leaving me deaf in the process), "How many times do I have to tell you? I hated Jane's flowers!"

Uh, okay.

I told them to try to keep it down while they figured it out.

They were both crying when I left.

-P.W.

Oregon

<u>Runaround Sue</u>

We had a new patient who obtained a nickname similar to 'Runaround Sue' from her fellow residents. She was a kind, attentive woman in her late-90s. She loved her makeup, was still very fashionable, and she was active…in several ways.

This patient was linked to an outbreak of an STD at our SNF. We found out she'd been seeing almost every man in our facility, and she had also had female partners.

I guess some residents had suspicions about this resident's behavior, but we found out that she swore her partners to secrecy. Eventually, a few of her partners leaked the secret, and good God, it got crazy.

For a while, our SNF was like a high school. We had screaming matches taking place in hallways, residents refused to speak to one another, and most of our residents divided into cliques. Some of our residents took to behaving like children. For example, Jane would speak, and then Joan would ask me, "Do you hear something? I could have sworn I heard the most annoying noise in the universe."

It became so ridiculous that we called in a relationship counselor. He spoke to residents privately and held group sessions in our game room for a month.

Thankfully, everything eventually went back to normal, but it was touch and go there for a while.

-S.B.

Idaho

Prozac for Paws

We had a woman come to our ER one afternoon. She was carrying a jewel-studded pet carrier that had her pet's name embroidered on it with golden thread.

I thought the woman was going to ask me how to get to a floor, but she leaned in and whispered, "Do you have a psychiatric ward for pets?"

I laughed at first, just because I thought she was joking.

I said, "I wish. I'd transfer up there in a heartbeat."

The woman didn't crack a smile. In fact, she looked royally pissed that I wasn't taking her seriously.

She said to me, "I didn't come here to be ridiculed. I came here because my Maltese is having serious self-esteem issues right now, and I think she needs help."

I just kind of looked at the woman for a second, and then my mouth started operating without a filter.   I blurted out, "What kind of self-esteem issues could a *dog* have?"

"For your information," the woman snapped, "she happened to receive the worst haircut of her life, and now she refuses to engage during her lunch dates. I've already called my attorney about filing a lawsuit against the groomer."

I decided right then and there that I didn't even want to get into it with the woman, so I apologized and told her that I was unaware of any hospital in our area that had a mental health unit for animals.

She sighed and thanked me for my time before she left.

-R.D.

Florida

Funny Florida

On my social media accounts, I will often dog on Florida for the outrageous news stories that come from the Sunshine State. It's all in good fun, I promise. You've probably heard me ask it before, but I can't help but ask again: Florida, you guys okay down there? Here are a few of my favorite wacky submissions from Floridan readers:

We went full lights and sirens to an apartment complex in the dead of night for a call from a frantic, crying caller who'd stated he was in desperate need of assistance. He stated he was 'trapped' in his apartment and told dispatch he was in 'serious danger' because he was positive he'd either 'have to rip it off and bleed to death,' or he'd be 'stuck forever and starve.' He told dispatch the code for his building and gave instructions for us to find a spare key hidden under a patch of loose carpet in the hallway.

We found the caller with his cell phone in his hand and his penis stuck in a hole in his bedroom door. He tearfully told us that he found a 'hot' video and wanted to 'try something new,' so he wanted to pleasure himself by inserting his penis into a hole he drilled through his bedroom door. I guess he didn't make the hole large enough, so he became stuck.

Fun times.

-J.L.

_____

I didn't ask how or why because I really didn't want to know. Afterall, it was Spring Break, and we were packed with tons of drunk, high, and/or just plain stupid patients.

This college-aged female's complaint was an odd one: she had a hermit crab stuck in her vagina and couldn't get it out because (and this is a direct quote), "It keeps pinching me when I stick my fingers up there."

I have no idea how, but the crab turned out to be perfectly fine and there was a rumor that someone from Lab eventually took it home as a pet.

-Y.T., P.A.

Back in the '70s, our rural newspaper ran an article about a vandalism spree that had plagued our small town. At the end of the article, the reporter said something like, "We may never find out who did this."

Someone sent a letter to the editor that basically stated, "I did it. Can you put my name in the paper?" The idiot gave us his full name, address, and his telephone number.

We called the police. They investigated, found the confession to be truthful, and they arrested the vandal. He got his wish; we ran his name in the paper in an article announcing that the criminal had been captured.

My supervisor came barreling out of his office with sweat dripping down his red face. I had never seen him look so embarrassed. Just a few seconds later, this absolutely stunning female applicant came walking out. She sheepishly apologized, and she left. I never really thought anything about it after that.

A few years later, after I had left the station, I went out for drinks with my former supervisor. He told me the story behind that moment.

When interviewing potential medics, he would say, "Tell me about one of your hidden talents." He always thought that added a fun aspect to the interview process.

Well, when he said that to the female applicant, he said she stood up and started stripping. She thought he was hitting on her, and she was so desperate for a job that she was prepared to do *anything*.

My former supervisor said he was so embarrassed for the woman and was so afraid that it would somehow become a legal issue that he ran out of the room. I had no reason to ever doubt the guy. He's been married to his wife for 40-something years, and he's always been the type who won't even *look* at another woman because he says he loves his wife.

-K.L.

A few years ago, we had this guy who came in for a week straight, several times per day, demanding drugs. He was clearly a drug seeker, and he had been flagged in our system by multiple practices for his antics. The most we felt we could offer him was Tylenol.

One night, he came in with his typical complaint of pain. I can't remember what he said hurt because his complaints were always inconsistent and often outlandish. When he was denied pain meds, he screamed at us (like usual) and stormed out.

He came back about an hour later, and he had a small alligator with him. I say 'small,' but the thing was probably two or three feet long. It was clearly a juvenile. I don't know where he got it, how he got it, or what exactly he planned to do with it. He stood in the lobby with the animal and screamed incoherent threats at us until security tackled him. We performed a soft lockdown of the emergency room lobby and left the alligator alone until the police came. The alligator was scared and just stayed in the corner, where it kind of watched everyone and would occasionally back up against the wall.

Someone said the man was charged with illegally possessing wildlife and was fined. I don't really know what happened to him. I think they took the alligator to a safe-release location.

-P.W.

We had a blind spot behind one of our in-network clinics. People knew there weren't cameras back there, so the lot would always be littered with needles, broken bottles, used condoms, and other disgusting items. The police patrolled the area and made a few arrests and/or wrote tickets, but people still came to our clinic to party on weekends and overnight. There were a few instances when we'd pull in on Monday morning and we'd find people passed out against the building.

Management decided to install cameras back there and hoped they'd act as deterrents for that type of behavior. Unfortunately, since there hadn't been cameras at the back of the clinic for years, nobody realized they were there.

Let me tell you what…The first few days (or nights, whatever) of footage was *crazy*! People were on camera having wild sex, shooting up and nodding out, dealing drugs, and my favorite…You could see police lights flashing in the distance, and then a man ran behind our building. He worriedly looked around for a few minutes, but once he realized the cops didn't know where he'd gone, he sat on the ground and started pulling tacos out of his pants (*not* his pockets—his pants!). It was clear he was probably having financial trouble, but I just thought it was hilarious that we would catch a taco thief on camera.

Some of the footage was so wild that we had to look away. We turned footage of violent crimes over to the police department.

Management *finally* put up several signs that warned that the lot was being monitored by security cameras, and the crazy happenings came almost to a full stop literally overnight.

-K.A.

We had to call for officer backup one night because our 'OD patient' had *clearly* not OD'd. He was running around the yard of his trailer almost completely naked (unless you count the crotchless female panties he had on), and when we approached him, he picked up a toad, grabbed my partner (she had bruises on her arms by the time we made it to the hospital), and tried to force the toad down her shirt. Luckily, I managed to push the patient away from my partner, and I stepped between the two, so he couldn't grab her again.

Right before we turned to go back to our bus, the patient bit into the toad. Most disgusting, disturbing thing I've ever seen in my entire career.

Officer backup arrived. The patient was tased, but it made little difference. They got the guy restrained, and we were all too happy to push some meds.

-P.J.

I retired a few years ago and went out with a bang. My last patient *ever* was a man in his 80s. His grandson called 911 because grandpa, a heavy drug user in the past, shot up bath salts. We found him in the backyard, naked, threatening to kill the family dog. We didn't feel that he posed a threat to us, so we brought him down, restrained him, and transported him to the ER.

About 10 to 20 years ago, we had a new mother who wanted to name her baby an offensive racial slur, pronounced and spelled the same. Thankfully, the patient's mother talked her out of it.

This is one of those situations where I can now laugh at the patient's behavior, but I can't laugh at the patient herself. She had to go off her meds during her pregnancy and she wasn't in the right state of mind.

I really don't know what would have happened if the patient's mom hadn't come to visit.

-Anonymous at request

I had to ask security to forcefully remove a female from my office one morning.

This female was in my office to apply for financial assistance or a full discharge of her recent ED bill.

When our accounting program determined that the female would not be eligible for a full discharge and instead would be eligible for a minor discount, she offered me oral sex in exchange for a full discharge.

As soon as I declined the female's offer, she *removed her dentures* and offered again. When I declined again, she tried to speak seductively, and she asked, "Are you sure?"

She became irate once I declined a third time, and she began knocking items off my desk.

-N.E.

<u>Silent Night</u>

My partner and I responded to a potential OD outside of a mall one Christmas night. When we arrived, it seemed obvious (to us) that the patient had appeared only to have drank too much. He was surrounded by crushed beer cans and still had a bottle of almost-empty bourbon in his hand.

The patient was out cold. We loaded him in back, bundled him up with blankets, and started transport. Since his vitals were okay at the time, my partner drove, and I sat up front.

All was well for a while. My partner and I were driving in silence on the way to the ER, since we'd both stupidly left our phones at the station and had no music to listen to (unless you counted the radio's non-stop Christmas music...no thanks).

We were almost sideswiped by a vehicle as we crossed through an intersection, and that made me jump a little bit. Whenever anything like that happens, the other car always seems to be coming at *my* side. I don't know if the universe is trying to threaten me or what, but it never gets less scary.

As soon as that came to pass, my partner and I returned to our silent night.

When we were about five minutes out from the ER, I started zoning out and just stared out the window at the blur of multicolored lights strung up on the houses we passed. It was eerily serene for a Christmas night, almost like we were just driving an empty bus around an empty world.

With no warning whatsoever, the patient in back sat up and screamed, "AHHHHHHHHHH!"

My partner was so startled that he swerved into oncoming traffic and was cussing up a storm. I was so caught off guard that it's quite possible that I peed myself a little bit. I don't want to confirm or deny anything publicly.

I whipped around in my seat and yelled back, "My dude, come on!"

I don't think he heard me because it appeared that he'd took to lying down again, and he was out cold.

When we gave report to the ER, we did not mention the patient's screaming episode. We considered mentioning it, but we thought it'd be a lot funnier if the ER staff experienced the patient in the same way we had. I did, however, mention the episode in my own report.

-F.R.

Ohio

Excuse Me, Pardon Me

My patient noticed his gown was defective, so I asked him to sit tight while I went to the supply closet for another gown. He was totally naked, so I figured he'd just cover himself with a sheet and wait in his room.

As I was digging through the supply closet, I heard a bunch of people gasping and making loud noises.

I peeked my head out to see my nude patient trying to secretly tiptoe around the nurses' station to get candy out of a glass jar that we had on the counter.

"John!" I shouted. "You know you're not supposed to be eating that!"

He stopped in his tracks, pouted, and then slowly walked back to his room.

I honestly don't know why he would try to sneak to the candy jar *naked*. About 20 nurses, doctors, patients, and family members had seen all John had to offer.

And really, the candies weren't even that great. Someone had gone to the supermarket and loaded up a paper bag of the 'buy this candy by weight' caramels and butterscotch discs. Not worth showing your ass to the entire ER, in my opinion.

-E.T.
Iowa

According to 12 reader submissions from the past six months, yes, patients *have* suffered injuries from creating the iconic leap scene from *Dirty Dancing.*

There may have even been *more* than 12; I haven't opened all my submissions yet!

Living My Best Life

When dispatch radioed at 01:15 and said we were the unit nearest to the call, my partner yelled out on a hot mic, "Bullllllshit."

That was strike one against us.

Dispatch also told us, "It should be an easy run. It's just a transport, so suck it up."

File that under, 'Lies dispatch tells.'

When we rolled up on scene, it wasn't too difficult to spot our patient. There was a woman lying in a mud puddle in 33-degree weather. She was wearing a bikini, and she looked like she was out like a light. A bunch of people were kneeling by her.

We couldn't park immediately because quite a scene was taking place along the curb and in the middle of the street. Two men were naked, shooting Roman candles at one another as they ran around like buffoons. We honked until they got out of the way. As I was parking, I just happened to look over and see another naked man in the window of the residence.

Yeah, still not entirely sure why so many people were naked. Not sure I want to know. Some things are better that way.

We grabbed the gurney and headed over to the chick we had been calling 'Bikini Barbara.'

"Did she take anything?" my partner asked.

A young woman looked at us like we each had three heads and then just shook hers.

"Did she hit her head?" asked my partner.

"No," the woman replied.

Already tired of playing 20 Questions, I got to the point and asked with a sigh, "Okay, then what's going on with her that you needed to call 911?"

"We didn't call 911," the woman said. "She just did a bunch of Fireball shots and passed out, so we were gonna carry her inside."

I muttered a few foul words and then asked, "Well, who called 911?"

The young woman shrugged and said, "You should go inside and talk to the people in there. They were lighting each other on fire earlier."

What the F kind of holiday party was this?!

Inside, things were even crazier than outside. People were having sex in the hallway. There were a few people snorting drugs in the living room. Two guys were setting off fireworks in the downstairs bathroom, and then the smoke alarm started going off. There were a lot of naked people there, but more were dressed than not. There had to have been about 50 people in the house.

We probably asked about 20 of the people, "Did you call 911?" before someone was able to say, "No, but I know who did."

This guy, who was walking around with a cookie sheet that was lined with about 50 pizza rolls, walked us to the kitchen. I noticed he wasn't letting anyone grab pizza rolls off the sheet. He'd apparently made 50 pizza rolls for himself and was just walking around with the entire pan.

The kitchen was where the real party was, I guess.

Our patient was sitting on the kitchen island. We could hardly see him because the huge plastic cheese balls jar was fogged up. Yes, his head was stuck inside it. Yes, that is why someone called 911. All the other crazy freaking things going on at that house, and someone called 911 because an idiot got his head stuck in a plastic jar.

"Yo," one of the guy's friends said, "911's here."

"911 is here," I agreed.

I walked over to the patient and lightly thumped on the jar.

"Why'd you do this, guy?" I asked.

When he spoke, his voice echoed.

"Ever seen *Mars Attacks!*?" he asked.

"Is that the ones with Jack Black?" I asked.

"Uh-huh," he replied.

"Yeah," I said. "I've seen it. Why'd you do this?"

The patient then just said, "Ack! Ack! Ack!" and started laughing so hard that he fell off the kitchen island.

His idiot friends were all laughing and taking pictures. We asked them to put their phones away because we didn't want to end up on some viral Facebook video. I'm sure there's a video of us floating around somewhere, though, because most of the people in the kitchen were anything but sober.

I had to hold the patient still while my partner used a pocketknife to carefully cut the jar, starting from the top to bottom. It allowed us to pull the jar in half. We had to use our shears to cut the rim from around his neck.

As soon as we got the rim off the guy's neck, he threw his hands in the air, screamed, "I'm living my best life!" and then he puked all over me. It was disgustingly obvious that he had consumed a large quantity of cheese balls before he stuck the jar on his head. I think he also ate some fries sometime that night, and I reeked of regurgitated beer.

I knew I didn't have any clothes in the ambulance, and I really didn't want to ride back to the station in puke clothes, so I took off both my shirts and was then half-naked in the kitchen. I started to feel like I was part of the party.

I'm not a young guy. Before I walked into that house, I thought I was doing okay for someone my age. My ego went from 'just okay' to 'really low' when a few of the young women in the room started making gagging noises and turning away. I work out four times a week, and I used to think I was in pretty good shape, but I guess I'm 'hairy' and 'hideous' and—yeah, my favorite: 'like, grandpa-old.' (I'm 43, by the way.)

One of the young women started arguing with her boyfriend, who then begrudgingly took off his overshirt and handed it to me. I would have rather had his plain white tee, but instead I was now wearing a shirt that made a dirty joke about the size of my penis.

I smelled like combination of an Axe Body Spray commercial and a weed dispensary, but at least I was no longer covered in puke.

Just when we thought it was over and we were walking out, a young woman at the top of the stairs yelled down, "Hey, are you 911?"

"Just say no," I told my partner…who was wearing a county 911 shirt.

We couldn't lie our way out of that one.

The woman complained, "We've been waiting, like, forever for you. Hurry up. I don't think she's breathing now."

Wait. What?

That's when my partner and I realized something was wrong with my radio. It wasn't working *at all*.

Yeah, the transport dispatch was for the patient we found upstairs, the college kid who'd drank so much that she passed out. I don't know what her friends were thinking, but they put her in a bathtub that was filled with ice and *salt*. The patient was not breathing, and her lips were blue.

I can't say too much more about that, but we called in a code to the nearest ER and got our butts there with that patient mighty quick.

Getting back to the rest of the confusion, allow me to explain. From what we learned from dispatch, the drunk patient's friends called 911 first, and *that* was supposed to be our 'easy' transport call. I guess dispatch considered it 'easy' because when the friends had called 911, the patient was still conscious and breathing. We had, instead, been directed to the kitchen to Cheese Ball, whose friends called 911 *after* we had arrived on scene. Dispatch swore up and down she radioed us and asked us to 'peek in' and see if we needed additional units on scene. A 'miscommunication' got us both off the hook for that, as management concluded that all patients involved were treated on scene. I must admit, I am still a bit frazzled about the condition of our ETOH patient. If I've learned anything from that night, it's to *always* check my radio on scene, even if I just checked it two minutes ago.

Oh, I've also learned to carry extra clothes.

-K.L.

Location withheld at request

<u>Never Seen That Before</u>

I'm probably going to Hell for laughing about this all these years later, but go big or go home, right?

We were transporting a psych patient to another facility. He was ambulatory and didn't seem to pose a threat to anyone, so we were just walking through the ER like no big deal.

A guy at the registration desk was telling the ER clerk that there was something wrong with his leg. I don't think she asked for this, but the patient reached up the leg of his shorts and popped off his prosthetic. He waved it in the clerk's face to show her a sharp piece or something.

My psych patient *flipped the heck out* and had a complete meltdown in the lobby.

He kept screaming, "He just pulled off his leg! He just pulled off his damn leg!"

He ran up to an old woman who was standing in line, and he screamed, "Did you see that? Oh my God, did you *see* that? He just ripped his own leg off!"

My guy was completely serious. He didn't seem to understand that the leg was a prosthetic. Totally blew his mind.

My partner and I had to convince our patient that the leg was fake. He insisted upon touching the prosthetic, so he could know for sure.

The patient at the desk thought it was hilarious, so no harm was done.

-Initials and location withheld at request

Fear

We responded to a 911 call placed by a frantic, incoherent man who basically screamed bloody murder during his entire call. Dispatch could basically make out his address and that he believed he was having a heart attack.

We walked by a floral arrangement and a few balloons on the front porch, entered the house, and found the patient curled behind his couch, holding a steak knife. I thought for sure he was high or something. He was trembling uncontrollably, and he had urinated.

He refused to allow us to transport him through the front door.

The patient was deathly afraid of balloons, so when he opened his front door to see the floral arrangement and three helium balloons, he spiraled into a panic attack.

We did transport him to the hospital. He was a mess, I'm telling you. I felt so bad for him because I've never, ever seen anyone with a phobia that severe before.

I did the guy a solid after we transported him, and I went back to his house to take the balloons off the flower basket and moved the arrangement to the side of the porch. I don't know how he functions out in the world. Poor guy.

-D.U.

Maine

I had to file a formal complaint against one of our traveling nurses because she stopped chest compressions during a code to step back and watch the ending of a reality show that was playing on the patient's television.

I really couldn't understand how she became so distracted by a TV show while our patient was dying.

-B.E.
Washington

__When Memes Come to Life__

S.C.-F. from Oregon sent in a conversation an ER physician and she had with a college-aged patient at 03:00.

RN: So, you came by ambulance for finger pain. Is that right?

Patient: Yeah.

RN: Did you injure yourself recently?

Patient: No.

RN: Your finger just started hurting?

Patient: No. Yeah. Well, kinda.

RN: Can you point to which part hurts?

Patient: Well, it really doesn't hurt right now.

RN: It doesn't hurt anymore?

Patient: No.

RN: So, you called 911, and then your finger stopped hurting?

Patient: Well, it only hurts if I move it a certain way.

RN: Okay. Do you think you can show me? If the pain becomes too much to bear, you can stop moving it, okay?

Patient: Okay.

The patient then sticks up his index finger and uses his other palm to bend his finger back towards the top of his hand.

Patient: Okay, now it's starting to hurt.

RN: Stop, stop. It only hurts when you do that?

Patient: Yeah.

RN: But otherwise, does it hurt?

Patient: No.

RN: *Mutters* You're kidding me.

RN: Hold on. I'm going to get the doctor.

Patient: Okay. Hey, do you think I'll have to get an X-ray?

RN: I doubt it, but just sit tight. I'm going to get the doctor.

Five minutes later...

Doctor: So, uh, the nurse just told me that your finger hurts when you move it a certain way.

Patient: Yeah.

RN: And you told me that it doesn't hurt unless you move it that way, right? (The RN explained to me that she entered the room with the physician because he did not believe her account of the patient encounter.)

Patient: Right.

Doctor: Can you show me? I know you just showed her, but I need you to show me.

The patient then repeated the action. This time, he pushed his finger back slightly more toward the top of his hand and screams.

Doctor: Are you serious right now?

Patient: Yeah. It really hurts when I do that.

Doctor: Uh, have you considered maybe *not* doing that?

Patient: Well, it's not supposed to hurt if I do that, right?

Doctor: Wrong. You're hyperextending your finger.

Patient: So, you're telling me it's supposed to hurt when I do that?

Doctor: *Mutters* Oh my God.

RN: Yes, it's supposed to hurt. Your body is trying to tell you not to do that.

Patient: Will all of my fingers hurt if I do that?

Doctor: *Shrugs* You're already in the emergency room. Go ahead and try.

The patient then did the same thing to three other fingers before he was told to stop.

Patient: Man, it really hurts when I do that.

Doctor: Then don't do that. Nurse, get him out of here, please.

The other night, one of our RNs called us (security) because she encountered a man in the parking lot. He was using a stick to beat against cars.

When we approached him, he suddenly pretended he was blind, and he held the stick like it was a cane.

"Not gonna work, buddy," I said to him.

Internally, I wanted to laugh my butt off. I don't know how he thought he'd get away with that.

He complained that we were abusing a disabled person, but he seemed to see just fine when we said we were calling the cops and he ran from us.

-C.L.

South Carolina

<u>Boy Toy</u>

We had an angry grandmother bring her grandson to our ED in the late afternoon. She said that when her grandson got off the bus after his day in Kindergarten, he was carrying a Barbie doll.

"Okay," I said slowly. Clearly, I wasn't following.

"Well," grandma snapped, "he's a boy. I think he might be gay."

"And what's the problem again?" I, a gay male, asked.

"I just told you. He was playing with a doll. He said his mom bought it for him. I think he's gay."

"Ma'am," I said with a sigh, "I'm honestly not following what the issue is. Is he hurt?"

"No," she said.

"Is he sick?" I asked.

She thought and then said, "I think he might be. Boys his age should be playing with trucks and soldiers and boy toys."

Inner me giggled a little. Outer me asked, "So, you want me to admit him to the ED because he...played with a Barbie?"

She nodded. "Mm-hmm," she said. "That's what I want. I think he needs to talk to a guidance counselor."

"Because he played with a Barbie?" I asked.

She nodded.

I didn't exactly have a choice in the matter, so I registered the child and as soon as the kid's name popped up on our electronic tracking board, someone came up to triage the patient in a little room to the side of our office.

I wasn't exactly eavesdropping, but I wasn't exactly trying to ignore the conversation, either. I tried my best to focus on my paperwork, but I couldn't help but to overhear the conversation.

After grandma explained the situation to the triage nurse, the nurse was quiet for about a full minute.

Finally, the triage nurse asked the child, "Why do you like playing with your Barbie so much?"

The boy hesitated, I guess, because I heard the nurse tell him it was okay to tell the truth, and that nobody would be mad at him.

"Why do you like playing with that doll?" asked his grandma.

This kid shouted excitedly, "Because she has boobies!"

I heard grandma then ask, "You *like* boobies?"

"Yeah!" the kid replied.

Grandma didn't say anything at first, but then I heard her say, "Well how 'bout that?"

She asked triage if they could leave without seeing a doctor, and since the nurse hadn't taken vitals or performed any sort of examination, nobody saw a reason why grandma couldn't leave with the boy. I marked them as LWBS (left without being seen).

I couldn't stop laughing, and neither could the triage nurse. I thought it was hilarious that this kid's grandma was so scared to think that his playing with 'girl toys' would make him gay, but it turned out to be something totally different (not saying you can't like boobies if you're gay). I honestly wanted to go back there and give the kid a high five before he left.

-P.W.
Alabama

We once transported a patient whose friend helped him carve, 'Marry me?' into his chest as a unique way to propose to his girlfriend, who was in nursing school.

Idiot covered up this huge wound with a rag, told his girlfriend he hurt himself, and said her he needed her to look at it to see if he should go to the hospital.

She told him he was an idiot, said she never planned to be with him long-term, and told him that yes, he should go to the hospital.

I heard they had a counselor come talk to him, just to evaluate his mental state for doing something like that in the first place.
Someone in the ER told me the counselor said he was 'balanced, just stupid.'

-K.W.
Ohio

What a Day

This submission was sent in pieces by members of the fire department, police department, emergency room staff, and EMS—one of the first of its kind. These submissions have been broken up so the story could be told in linear fashion.

G.K. of the police department writes:

We received a frantic call directly to our station from a clerk at a used car dealership. She stated that upon arriving to the lot that morning, she found a note taped to the front door that stated multiple bombs had been planted in and near the building. The note also stated that the lot employees were being watched off-the-clock, and evidence would suggest this was true. Our subject had included a photograph of another lot clerk picking up her children at preschool.

Our officers advised the caller to remain calm, move away from the building and property, and wait for responders to arrive.

U.D. from the fire department writes:

Shortly after arriving on scene, our guys found three suspicious packages strategically placed around the building's perimeter. We notified officers of our findings, and the residences and businesses adjacent to the car lot were evacuated as a precaution. A window had been busted out of the back of the building, and just by doing a quick peek inside, it was clear that the subject had placed two more packages inside.

After some time and after saying many prayers, we concluded that none of the five boxes contained explosives or explosive components. Three of the five boxes contained bricks and packing peanuts. The other two boxes contained what I can only best describe as junk: old cords, pens, used notepads, and similar items.

We gave the all-clear and let officers take over from there.

G.K. continues:

It was not incredibly difficult to find our subject. For starters, the subject had written the threatening note on a personalized notepad, so we had a first name. The evidence that broke the case however, happened to be the 'bombs' themselves. Four of the five boxes had been shipped from the same online retailer and still had shipping labels affixed to their exteriors. Our subject's full name and shipping address were printed on every label.

The car lot employees worked with us to provide clues as to what might have caused the subject to threaten the business. We discovered that the subject had recently purchased a 'buy here, pay here' vehicle. The subject had made a small down payment and had agreed to make weekly payments in excess of $100 to the car lot. If the subject failed to comply with the sales contract, the car lot was within its rights to repossess said vehicle.

According to the lot owners/employees, the subject had contacted the office multiple times to state that the payment no longer worked for the family, as 'they only had extra money during tax time.' The subject stated he would not be paying his next weekly installment, and he allegedly threatened an employee over the phone. That exchange had taken place only a few days prior to the bomb threat, according to the lot owners.

According to lot employees, the subject was informed that his vehicle would be impounded 'on or around' the date the bomb threat had been called in to our station.

We wasted no time and/or resources when we dispatched units to the subject's residence. Based on the nature of the incident, we had reason to believe that the subject was possibly armed and/or dangerous.

Officers spotted the subject fleeing from his residence after jumping from a second story window. He landed on a patio table and attempted to run from the scene. Once officers caught up with the subject, he was combative and resisted arrest. It was at this time that he stabbed one of our officers in the eye with a neon plastic sword-shaped swizzle stick that he'd apparently been keeping in his pocket. Our officer deployed pepper spray, but the subject managed to get away.

We notified dispatch of the need for medical transport for one of our officers, and right around this time, our K9 unit arrived nearby. The K9 officer was released to bring down the subject. The subject was bitten, but then he twisted the dog's leg and left our K9 injured. The subject then hopped a fence. Due to its injuries, our K9 unit was unable to follow.

The subject was met by additional patrol on the other side of the fence, and at this time he was tased. He not only busted his face open when he did a dead-fall to a pile of discarded chunks of concrete, but he also urinated and defecated himself.

M.R. from EMS details:

I was one of two EMS units dispatched on scene. My coworkers had already loaded an injured female officer for transport to the nearest ED. According to radio reports, the officer experienced mild bleeding and reported temporary blindness stemming from the puncture to her eye.

My patient was handcuffed and lying on his side when I arrived. He was attempting to remove his jeans. The patient was screaming obscenities and threats against law enforcement. He kept talking about how he had been ripped off by a car lot, and he shouted that he would kill everyone involved with his arrest, treatment, and repossession of his car, should it be repossessed.

Though the patient complained of chest and facial pain, he wouldn't shut up for half a second. He refused to let me treat his facial injuries. The patient smelled of diarrhea and urine. I also detected methamphetamine residue from the patient and alerted officers to this detail that they had seemingly overlooked during the commotion.

The patient bit through my glove and broke skin. He swallowed a chunk of my flesh and promptly vomited. I bandaged my hand the best I could while officers assisted my partner in loading the patient. Two officers accompanied my partner and me to the ED. On the way to the ED, I was instructed by my supervisor to complete the run and to then register as a patient for my injuries.

At the ED, an RN irrigated my wound and advised I monitor the bite for tissue devitalization.

Officer G.K. continues:

We received a search warrant for the subject's residence due to the nature of his initial threats against the car dealership and its employees. While we searched the residence for explosives and explosives components, we found a meth lab set up in an extra bedroom. In the bedroom was also a child's playpen and toys. It was clear that a child had recently been in the room, as there were used diapers on the floor. It was unclear to us where the subject's family was. Additional meth lab components were located in the subject's basement and garage. He had a great number of chemicals and items that could have been used in the making of bombs, had he actually followed through with his threat against the car lot.

We notified dispatch of a need for the fire department's RIT unit (Rapid Intervention Team), and as a precaution, we asked nearby neighbors to evacuate.

While our team worked with nearby law enforcement to dismantle the meth lab, the subject's wife and two children returned to the residence. The wife attempted to flee from the scene, but quick-thinking members of the fire department detained her until officers could intervene. The wife and both children displayed physical markers of exposure to methamphetamine and chemicals used in manufacturing methamphetamine.

One would *think* a mother would want to go peacefully, since her children were present, but this was simply not the case whatsoever. The mother attempted to use her youngest child as a human shield, thus preventing officers from physically apprehending her. Both children were crying while their mother shouted at officers and firefighters. Neighbors who'd evacuated were standing down the block on their neighbors' lawns, watching the whole ordeal. It was a disaster.

We finally convinced the mother to release her children and come peacefully. Her compliance lasted approximately 30 seconds. Luckily, the children were in the hands of an officer and firefighter. Their mother headbutted an officer and broke his nose. She complained of a headache and chest pain, so it was no surprise that she demanded to receive medical attention before being processed in our facility. CPS was notified, and the children were transported by law enforcement to the nearest ER.

S.R. and Y.Y.-Z. of the emergency room write:

Our first patient received from this debacle was a female officer presenting with ocular trauma. She complained of temporary blindness while en route, but upon arriving at our facility, she stated her eyesight was only minorly disturbed. An examination concluded that the patient would not require surgery or extensive treatment. She was treated and discharged.

A male medic was treated for an occlusion bite to his hand. Human bites require extensive cleaning and irrigation to (hopefully) avoid future infection. Because the patient was a first responder, we felt confident that he would recognize the signs of infection, should one occur. There was little we could offer the patient elsewhere.

Our third patient from the scene was an adult male with a six-inch laceration from his nose to his chin. The wound required light debridement and irrigation prior to requiring sutures. The patient also complained of chest pain, but an examination concluded that the patient's heart was working 'just right.' Though two officers accompanied the patient to our ER, we required the assistance of our security team. The patient was restrained during the duration of his ER admittance. During his time in our ER, he verbally assaulted many members of our staff.

Another officer arrived a few hours later. He had sustained a broken nose during an altercation with a combative patient. He had already 'set' his own nose and stated he was simply following department procedure by registering as a patient.

Two children between the ages of one and five were transported to our ER by law enforcement. An employee from Social Services met with the children. Examinations suggested the children were malnourished, dehydrated, and had been exposed to methamphetamine. Both children presented contusions and/or trauma consistent with abuse, both physical and sexual.

An adult female was brought in by law enforcement. She complained of head pain and chest pain. Following examinations, the patient was provided a dose of NSAIDs and was transported to jail.

During this time, our registrar department alerted us of a visitor. The woman identified herself as the grandmother of the two children. She became unruly and boisterous when she was approached by a Social Services employee. Security was required to remove the visitor from our lobby. Someone called police after the woman used a landscaping brick to break off a side mirror of an ambulance that was parked in front of our ER. The woman fled before officers arrived.

G.K. concludes:

Our subject and his wife were obviously arrested. We were notified of damage to property, but we were unable to find the subject once we arrived on scene. However, the female was later apprehended after she was caught shoplifting cough syrup at a nearby pharmacy. Two others were arrested in relation to manufacturing and distribution of the original subjects' meth lab. The children involved were placed with a foster family until the involved parties could receive an order from family court.

I began that day at 02:30. I couldn't sleep for crap, and I remember begging, "Please don't let anything wild happen today." You can see how that turned out.

Our department and the FD worked well past sundown to secure the location of the meth lab. It took some time to write the reports up on the day's events, so I don't think I got home and in bed until after midnight. I thought my wife was going to kill me because I had missed our anniversary reservation because of this mess. She was incredibly forgiving.

Our K9 officer made a swift recovery from a sprained paw. Our department and others in the community gifted his handler with treats and toys to aid in recovery.

-Location withheld

The funniest call of my career had to be a report of an unconscious patient lying on a city sidewalk (which is nothing new around here, believe you me).

According to bystanders, the patient had rushed down a flight of stairs and attempted to leap into a bus before the bus driver closed the doors.

The patient ran face-first into the closed doors and was KO'ed in an instant.

I'm probably going to hell for laughing at this, but I think the best part was that the bus driver didn't even wait. I can only imagine that the driver shrugged and drove away.

Patient was fine, by the way.

-K.A.
New Jersey

Important Reminder

A few years ago, my family and I vacationed down in Florida, where we'd rented a house. It was my family (me, my husband, two kids, and a dog), my brother, my two sisters and their husbands (along with one child and another dog), and my mother and father.

We had a wonderful time in Florida before it was finally time to pack up and make the trip home. My family drove off in all directions. At the time, I lived in Southern Indiana, my brother lived in Northern Indiana, my sisters lived in Ohio and Kentucky, and my parents lived in Nebraska. We told each other to text, call, or email once we each made it home okay.

Unfortunately, my brother was involved in a nasty accident that left him severely injured and another driver deceased. I've since made peace with the fact that the other driver chose to drive while impaired. What's done is done, and I don't like to hold grudges.

My brother was transferred to many hospitals, saw so many doctors that I couldn't keep count, and my parents pushed specialists to try everything under the sun, until their own funds were exhausted. It was of no use. Each and every doctor explained that my brother suffered from a traumatic brain injury. He would never be able to speak, bathe himself, eat on his own, walk, or basically do any of the things that we do everyday and take for granted. Essentially, he would be forced to spend the rest of his life in a bed, hooked to machines, dependent on nurses. My parents had my brother admitted to an LTC facility, and just from what I'd seen during visits, they took great care of him and treated him well.

Stress and cancer caught up to my parents. My father died from lung cancer, and then my mother died two weeks later. Their deaths came just a few months following my brother's admittance to the LTC facility. It was a rough year for all of us. We had my parents cremated per their wishes. My sisters took over my parents' house and their belongings.

My parents' will/trust wanted all remaining funds to be left to my siblings and me to cover my brother's healthcare expenses so none of us would have to worry about it for a while. I say none of us, but honestly, it all fell on my shoulders because my sisters wanted no part in it. That comes off harshly, but I'm not angry, and I completely understand why they did not wish to be responsible for my brother's care.

I called the LTC and they had me come in for an appointment with a counselor person, where they made me the emergency contact for my brother. We changed all information to my name. I worked with lawyers, banks, and the facility to transfer funds. It took a while, and it was tiresome.

Life got in the way, so I didn't visit as frequently as I'd hoped. We moved, the kids started new schools, and the dog ran away and was missing for three weeks at one time (someone had picked her up, thinking she was a stray, so she spent three weeks eating canned food and chilling with a guy who took her boating until he took her to the vet for grooming and they scanned her microchip— No ill feelings; he just honestly didn't think to have the dog scanned first.). It was hectic, and I didn't visit for at least six months at one point. I don't think my brother would have wanted me to regret that, so I try not to.

I returned from work and noticed a vivid sheet of paper sticking out from my door. It had written on it that the postman could not deliver a package because nobody was home to sign. My husband's birthday was that weekend, and I had been expecting a $2,000 gaming computer set up to arrive. I kept thinking to myself, 'Crap, crap, crap!' at the idea that he'd find out that I'd ordered it and he'd somehow get to it first. I had 15 minutes to get to the post office before it closed, so I raced there and signed for this 'package' that was really just an envelope with correspondence inside.

The first line was, "We regret to inform you…"

My brother had passed away two days earlier. My brother DIED, and they MAILED ME A LETTER!

I was so mad. I was hurt. I had feelings I couldn't even explain. How *dare* they tell me in a letter *after* my brother died!

The contact at the LTC let me scream and cry for a few moments, but then she said to me, "Sherry, let me read back the number we have for you, okay?"

She did, and my heart dropped right out of my chest.

She read me my *old* phone number. I glanced over at the envelope through tears and realized that the envelope had my *old* address on it. I think the only reason it got to me is because I knew someone who'd worked at the old post office, and she was still putting in forwarding information for me on things I'd forgotten to change, like magazines and things that you have to change manually.

The LTC said they'd even sent a sheriff to my old home on the night my brother passed because they couldn't reach me by phone, but the new occupants didn't know who I was. A quick call to the sheriff's officer confirmed the LTC contact's account. It was my fault. I never updated the number on the NOK section.

I apologized 10 million times and 10 million ways to the LTC contact. She apologized too. We cremated my brother and had a nice service the following week. We spread his ashes with my parents' ashes during our next trip to Florida, just because I think that's where we were the happiest as a family.

I've stop beating myself up about this. I try to keep negative energy out of my life, and I try to let it go if it enters my thoughts. I must admit, I think of this from time to time and still feel guilty.

This wasn't meant to be a sad story, and I hope nobody feels sorry for me or my family because that's not what I stand for. I do wish, though, that you'd remind people to keep contact information up to date, especially with places like LTCs, nursing homes, or even hospitals in case of emergencies.

-S.F.-K.
Indiana

Tonight, I realized how stupid my new partner is.

We arrived on scene for an injured child, and there were dogs stopped at the edge of the driveway, just barking.

The patient's mom said to us, "Don't worry, we have an invisible fence."

My partner deadass asked her, "Oh, okay. So, do I have to, like, jump over it, or is there a gate somewhere?"

She, the patient's father, and I just kind of looked at him, amazed at how someone could be so dumb.

I don't think he's gonna last long.

-C.C.

Indiana

<u>Biggest Regret</u>

I volunteer my time to sit with hospice patients and nursing home residents. Most of the patients I visit don't have friends or family. Sometimes, it's because they're the last living out of their friends and family. Other times, sadly, it's because they are either not on good terms with their loved ones, or they're overlooked in their time of need.

I was spending time with John, who was 103-years-old. I am not exactly sure how we ended up on the topic, but we were talking about living life to its fullest. We somehow began discussing our regrets. My biggest regret had been not pursuing my degree in art restoration. It had always been a passion of mine, and I think I would have been happier choosing that as a career, rather than entering early childhood development.

John scoffed at me and said, "Yeah? That's nothing."

I asked, "What's your biggest regret?"

Without skipping a beat, John replied, "I turned down a date with Jane B. because Joan C. was putting out. Broad gave me gonorrhea! And you know what? Jane B. ended up winning the lottery a few years later. Could've been a stay at home husband if I would've kept my willy in my pants."

I laughed until my sides hurt.

-D.E.
Colorado

<u>Neighbor from Hell</u>

My 12-year-old retriever underwent surgery to remove a cancerous tumor and had a sizeable incision on her side. I placed her on a pile of blankets I had spread out on the couch. She was still loopy from anesthetic, and while the direct causation was not funny, the faces she was making were funny. I decided to whip out my cell phone and capture a video to share on my Facebook page, since my children grew up with this dog and could not be with her due to college and work responsibilities.

While I was capturing my dog's funny faces, she accidentally rolled off the couch. Again, the causation wasn't funny, but seeing how she just lopped herself off the edge of the couch made me chuckle. I immediately ended the recording, placed my dog back on the couch, checked her sutures, and sat with her to keep her safe and comfortable.

I posted the video on my Facebook and explained that she had surgery that morning. Most of the comments were what I would expect, apologies and well wishes. I was grateful so many people were concerned for her wellbeing.

My next-door neighbor, Jane, had to be the party pooper. She posted under the video, "Not funny! You are a horrible human being. Maybe if you took better care of your pets, this one wouldn't have had to get surgery! I'm filing a police report for animal cruelty, and I've reported you to Facebook for spreading videos of animal abuse."

I put a laughing emoji as a reply and left it long enough for her to see it, and then I deleted that crazy bat from my friends list. Anyone who knows me or my family also knows that my dogs have been fed a raw diet from the time they were puppies. They're exercised daily. With the kids out of the house, my dogs now have their own bedroom, complete with a queen-size bed for them to sleep on at night. They're not only spoiled rotten, but they've been well cared for over the years. Unfortunately, cancer sometimes happens. There's nothing that can be done about that. I took no offense to my neighbor's rants because she was clearly one of those nutcases who wanted to assume what kind of life I provided for my dog from viewing a 20-second clip on social media.

Shortly after this mess, my radio went off. A fire had been called in about a block from my house. I am a volunteer firefighter and felt it necessary to respond since I was so close. I gated my dog in the kitchen. She was breathing well and responding well. She had gotten up twice to find a more comfortable place to sleep. I saw no reason not to leave her alone since my wife was due home from work soon.

When I arrived at the address on the radio, there was no fire. There wasn't even a structure on the lot for there to be a structure fire. I called in the information to the department and headed home.

My garage door was open when I arrived. At first, I thought I had left the door open by accident. Upon closer investigation, I realized the door leading from the garage to my mud room was also ajar. I conceal carry, but I did not have my firearm on me. I grabbed a claw hammer from my tool kit and cautiously entered the house.

Kid you not, Jane was in my kitchen, trying to coerce my dog to get up and leave with her. When I confronted her about being in my house, she became violent and tried to attack me with a cookie sheet. She managed to get one good blow to my head. The sheet wasn't one of those cheap ones, so it hurt and left me temporarily disoriented. I felt a tickle on my face and realized I was bleeding. Then I heard a yelp, and I realized I had stepped on my dog's tail.

Jane was still screaming about how I abused my pets when my second dog, a 230-pound St. Bernard, leapt over the gate that closed off the kitchen from the dining room, and he bit Jane on the arm. Coincidentally, that dog is named Cujo (my daughter, an avid horror flick fan, named the dog), and the name never really fit his personality until that incident.

I was able to call 911 and stay on the line until help arrived. Jane was arrested for breaking and entering. She was also charged with misinforming because *she* had called in a fake fire, just so she could have an opportunity to steal my dog. I was transported to the hospital because I felt woozy. The doctor said I was okay, but he advised me to go home and get some rest. He said sometimes you can just get hit hard enough or in the right spot to take you out, and boy, I think he was right.

My girl passed away a few months ago. Statistics said that dogs who have those types of masses removed only live a few months to a year afterward. She lived for six more months. It's not as long as we had hoped to have with her, but I think it was longer than she would have lived with the tumor, so I am grateful to have had the time with her.

My wife and I petitioned for a restraining order against Jane. She was not allowed to step foot on our property or contact us in any way.

Get this: She didn't end up getting jail time from what she did that day, just a fine and probation. I think it's just a tad bit funny that you can break into someone's house, beat them senseless with a household object, call in a false report, and *still* just get a slap on the wrist. But hey, I guess that's why we have the right to vote, yeah?

-D.W.
Ohio

Happy Birthday

I went out for my tenth 29th birthday in a row and possibly had a bit too much to drink. My husband walked me to the restroom, and I assured him that yes, I *could* manage to pee on my own.

I remember all the stalls being occupied, and I remember *really* having to pee. I had the bright idea to hoist myself up and pee in the sink. I wouldn't ordinarily do something like that, but Jose Cuervo would.

The sink fell off the wall while I was peeing. I hit my head when I fell, and then I tried to stand and fell into one of the pipes that had broken away from the wall. I didn't even feel the pipe on my head, but I knew I was bleeding. Water was going all over, and I couldn't stop peeing.

A few women came out of the stalls and just kind of stared at me. Someone ran out to find help, and that's when my husband came in.

He had to drive me to the ER (where I work), and I had to get two staples.

This happened *years* ago, but my husband is never gonna let it go. Every year since then, when we go out, he makes me use the buddy system to go to the bathroom.

-M.P.
Nevada

<u>Learn Something New</u> <u>Every Day</u>

Y.R. from Illinois sent in her recollection of an interesting call to 911:

Operator: 911, what's your emergency?

Caller (A female who sounded like she was in her 30s): Um, yeah, I just came outside to smoke, and I think I need you to send that guy who does the wildlife stuff.

Operator: What seems to be the problem, ma'am?

Caller: I think I found a new species. I need someone to come out and look at it. You know, just in case it's dangerous.

Operator: A new species of what?

Caller: I don't even know what it is, but it's hanging out of the tree in my front yard.

Operator: Uh, can you describe it to me?

Caller: A snake, maybe? I've never seen anything like it before.

Operator: A snake?

Caller: I don't know. It's really long and wiggling. And it's slimy.

Operator: It's slimy?

Caller: Yeah.

Operator: What color is it?

Caller: Uh, like a brownish color? I don't know, really. It's really gross. It kind of has spots on it.

Operator: Okay.

Caller: It looks like it's, like, twisted around itself. I don't know. I don't want to get too close to it. Like, what if it's something that came here from Australia or Scotland or something? Like, what if it bites me or something, and I die?

Operator: Ma'am, are you sure you're not looking at two slugs?

Caller: Slugs? Oh, you mean those snail things that don't have shells?

Operator: Yes, ma'am. That's what a slug looks like.

Caller: Well, I think it's a new species. I've never seen a slug look like this. I mean, it's really long, and it's just hanging from a branch by this slimy stuff. I really think you need to send someone out right away.

Operator: Ma'am, I think I know exactly what's going on.

Caller: How? Have other people seen these things? Should I keep my kids inside if these things are out here?

Operator: Ma'am, it sounds like you're describing slugs mating.

Caller: Mating? Like having sex?

Operator: Yes, ma'am.

Caller: Are you messing with me? Like, people shouldn't be made fun of when they call for help.

Operator: No, ma'am, I'm not messing with you. That's how slugs mate. I see them all the time on my trees out back.

Caller: So, they're just doing it, right here in my front yard?

Operator: That's what it sounds like, ma'am.

Caller: Are they dangerous?

Operator: Not as far as I know. It sounds like you have the typical garden slugs there.

Caller: Will you call that guy out here? I just need to make sure. Like, if it's something new that nobody's ever seen before, I don't want to be patient zero or whatever. And I have kids, too, so if it's really two slugs doing it, he should probably take these things away from here. I can't let my kids see this. They're not old enough to know about sex.

Operator: Uh…

Caller: Yeah, just go ahead and send him out here. I'm not gonna be able to sleep if you don't send the guy out here.

Y.R. states, "I wasn't going to call a conservation officer out at midnight, so I dispatched an officer to the caller's location. He confirmed that the caller was looking at slugs mating, and he assured the caller that she had nothing to fear."

If you're going to show up at 03:30 to bail your friend out of jail, PLEASE put some clothes on and be sober, for the love of God.

Yeah, woman came to bail her friend out. She was naked (only carrying a purse), and it was clear she was high.

She was also arrested for multiple charges that included public indecency, driving with a suspended license, driving impaired, and resisting a peace officer.

-D.M.
New York

Tales from Beyond

I receive plenty of submissions about the supernatural. Some readers do not particularly enjoy these submissions, but others do. Here are a few accounts from first responders and healthcare workers:

I was conducting a routine patrol of a warehouse during my overnight shift. When I pulled around to the side lot, I noticed a man trying to break into the building. I placed my vehicle in park, got out, and cautiously approached him.

At first, I thought the subject was going to comply with my orders. He placed his hands where I could see them, and he began to lower himself to his knees.

As I neared, the subject whipped around and assaulted me. I don't really know how it happened, really, because I have undergone extensive training. Still, the subject managed to knock my firearm out of my hands. At that point, I was more concerned with the possibility of this man getting my gun and either shooting me or another person with it. As I scrambled to grab my firearm, the subject kicked me in the abdomen.

I was six weeks pregnant and I had not announced my pregnancy to anyone yet—not even my boyfriend. I had planned to make the announcement a few days later, both to my department and also my family.

I became paralyzed with fear. My ex and I got divorced because a doctor told me I would never be able to conceive. I had been heartbroken since hearing that news, and I had given up on my dreams to have a child. I was so scared that something was going to happen to the baby and that I would never be able to get pregnant again that I couldn't force myself to move away from the subject.

This man kicked my gun out of reach, and he was able to pin my arms to the ground with one of his hands. He tore at my clothes and tore my blouse open. There was no doubt in my mind that he was going to attempt to rape me.

I was fighting as hard as I could, but the subject seemed to anticipate my every move. I was scared to death. Like I said, I am a trained officer. I didn't think I would have a problem with a man of this size, but I was struggling.

The subject started punching me when he saw that I had pressed my radio to call for help. Right before he punched me a third time, I heard something that sounded like an animal.

I glanced over and could have *sworn* that my dog was standing there, snarling at the subject. The dog looked identical to mine, right down to a distinct marking on its chest. This animal moved in slowly, taking calculated steps as if giving the subject an opportunity to do the right thing. Then, the dog barked.

I'd know that bark anywhere. My dog never, ever shut up. He barked at the wind, barked when he passed gas, barked at the TV, barked if someone knocked on a front door in China.

The problem with all this was that my dog had died a year earlier. He was old. He just fell asleep one afternoon, and he never woke up.

As the subject became more worried about this dog than what he planned on doing to me, I had the opportunity to not only get away from the subject, but also reach my firearm. As I was radioing for assistance, I quickly scanned the area for the dog. It was nowhere to be found. The subject even made a comment about how the dog seemed to be there one second, but it was gone the next.

I was sent to the hospital to get checked out, and everything was fine. I had some bruising for a while, but that was the least of my worries.

-T.H.
Washington

John had been with our station for decades. He and I had pretty much become great pals, family really. We often invited each other over for family events and backyard cookouts.

John learned he had cancer in Summer, and he died in the Fall. It took us all by surprise. We dedicated one of our new trucks to John, and all the guys chipped in to purchase a memorial bench. We had a metal nameplate engraved with his name, and we put the bench out back. John used to go back there all the time, just to clear his mind.

We were called to a structure fire one night. When we arrived on scene, we knew the residence would be a total loss. Most of the house was up in flames.

Out front, a crowd of neighbors formed a human barrier around a screaming woman. She was fighting tooth and nail, screaming that one of her daughters was still inside. She had carried her two youngest children outside first because they were nearest. She thought she had time to go back in for her other daughter.

The guys and I knew we had to think quick. We felt that it would be safest to go in through the window. It was clear where the child was, and we already knew that probably one of the only things saving this child was that her bedroom door was closed. It was the only room that didn't have flames shooting out from the busted windows.

We literally played rock, paper, scissors to make a choice, but the guy who lost was still kind of green for what this could entail. I decided to be the one to go inside. But once I got in through the bedroom window, I couldn't find the child. There was so much smoke flooding in from the vents and from the gap under the bedroom door that I could barely see my own hands. I kept tripping over toys and furniture, kept running into walls. I called out to the guys that the girl wasn't in her bedroom. They told me to come out, but I couldn't just leave a child in the house to die.

Against better judgment, I opened the child's bedroom door and flames came rushing in. It spread quickly. I heard coughing from a room that was separated from the child's bedroom by another door. I raced into that room and at first, all I could see were a bunch of toys. I noticed there was a small child hiding behind a play kitchen set, and I rushed over to her and tried to keep her calm. She continued to cough and started wheezing.

We couldn't go out through the door I'd just entered, and I didn't know how any of this would pan out. The child's bedroom was engulfed and either a beam or some part of the child's door frame had fallen over the doorway. And even if I tried sprinting through the room, I didn't know that I or the child would be able to exit the residence.

I started having my first on-scene breakdown. Of all the scenes I'd been to, of all the things I'd ever witnessed…This was it. This was the one I couldn't handle. This house was literally falling around me. The room I was in was now filled with thick, black smoke. The child had grown from hysterical to gasping for air. Flames started coming in from the door that separated her bedroom and the playroom. I panicked.

I don't know if this was my brain playing tricks on me, or if it really happened, but it felt real.

I saw John standing in the doorway between the room we were in and the child's bedroom, motioning for me to follow him. He said to me, "You gotta move now, Fred."

"I don't think I can get through all that," I called out. "It's too far gone."

He shook his head and said, "It's not a flashover yet, just looks like one."

I argued with him, "The door. I can't go through the door. There's something—."

He interrupted calmly, "It's not blocking you in. You gotta move now, Fred."

I knew if I didn't do *something* this child and I would both die there. So, I listened to John, and I ran through the doorway. Most of the room was on fire, but there was a narrow path that led us straight out the window. I handed off the child, and I got out of there. I don't think it was even 10 more seconds before flames shot out.

I told a few guys that I'd seen John inside. They seemed supportive, but I could tell they didn't believe me. When I mentioned the incident to my doctor, he told me I had probably imagined John being there to guide me as a coping mechanism, almost like my brain jumped into emergency mode because my nerves had swallowed me whole.

I still don't know if I imagined all this, or if John was really there. All I know is that it'd honestly make a lot of sense either way. The body does some crazy things when it's under pressure, but if I ever saw John's ghost someplace, I'd expect to see it on scene because he had dedicated his entire life to helping others.

I don't like how people look at me like I'm crazy, so I just don't bring it up anymore.

-F.L.

Location withheld at request

I work on a Peds ICU. My patient was between the age of six and eight. He was honestly a good child, but he liked to tell lies. For example, he spilled applesauce all over his sheets one day, and he said the doctor did it. Another time, he kept pressing his call button and told us that he didn't do it; he said there was a ninja in his room.

It was around 02:30 when I heard a television playing loudly. I tracked the racket to the patient's room. The television was turned to a channel that was playing cartoons, and the volume was almost up as high as it would go.

I scolded the boy and told him it was time for bed. He told me that he wanted to sleep, but he couldn't because the other boy wanted to watch TV. Because the patient was alone in the room, I brushed it off as him telling another lie. I thought maybe he was afraid to be alone that night, even though he had been in that room alone for three nights and hadn't had an issue yet.

"Well," I said, "tell your friend he needs to go to bed, too."

A few minutes later, as I was catching up on stocking our carts, I heard the TV again.

I went back to the room, told the patient he needed to go to bed, and then sighed when he told me, "It wasn't me. It was the other boy."

"You need to go to sleep," I said. "You're going to start waking up other kids if you keep it up."

The boy tried to argue with me about how *he* hadn't done anything. The other boy this, the other boy that.

"Go to sleep," I said to the patient.

I then unplugged the TV from the wall, and I left the room.

I don't even think it was five minutes later that I heard the TV. It was even louder than before.

"How did you reach the outlet?" I asked the patient. "Did you climb up on the table?"

He shook his head and said, "I didn't do it. The other boy did it."

I didn't believe him, but I also didn't know how he could have physically plugged the TV back in, especially since he had lines running every which way.

"You are the only boy in this room," I said. "Now, if you're scared, that's okay. You can tell me, and I can stay with you until you fall asleep."

He took that accusation personally and told me, "I'm not! It was the other boy. It was the boy with the big mark on his face. He said he wants to watch TV because I look like John. I told him my name is Jack."

My heart stopped for a good two seconds.

A few months earlier, we had a patient admitted to our floor following an accident. The child had a distinctive birthmark on his face. I can't go into detail, but that child passed away. He had died in that same room. He had a younger brother, probably around my patient's age, named John. John had a disability and wasn't always 'in the moment' with us. John's family would position his wheelchair between the window and the bed, and he would watch TV when his family came to visit his brother.

There was absolutely no way this child could have known about the deceased patient or that child's family. Nobody on our unit would *ever* discuss a child dying under our care, *especially* to another peds patient.

When I walked out of the room, I heard my patient grumble, "You're getting me in trouble."

I called for a float to stay with the patient until he fell asleep. She didn't report anything unusual. Every now and then, the TV in that room still turns on. I know I'm not crazy because other staff on the unit have reported it.

I feel uneasy about the idea that our unit (or any other) could have spirits walking around, so when the TV acts up, I force myself to believe that it's the wiring or something.

-E.G.

North Carolina

We had a patient come in who'd looked like she'd been to Hell and back. She had been involved in a crime spree and came to us with critical injuries, including stab wounds and an untreated gunshot wound.

This patient was the worst patient I've ever encountered. It was odd, too, because her vitals suggested she was knocking on death's door, but her behavior suggested otherwise. She fought everyone, physically and verbally. She bit, kicked, screamed, rubbed her excrement on staff, insulted everyone. It was horrible.

What's even stranger is what happened when the patient's family came to visit. Everyone who'd known her before said something to the effect of, "That's not the woman we know." The patient's behavior became worse when her family came around, so they agreed that until we could figure out what was wrong and she could heal from her injuries, they should not visit.

We had to restrain the patient and keep pumping her full of meds to keep her poor behavior at a minimum. I'd never seen a patient quite like her. Looking back, yes, I would say this patient reacted *exactly* like that little girl did in that possession movie. This woman's behavior was just outrageous, and I worked on Mental Health for 13 years, so I know what I'm talking about when it comes to witnessing outrageous behavior.

The patient coded, and I was the first in the room. It was really strange because out of nowhere, while all the sensors were going wild, she started thrashing around and screaming things I couldn't understand. Gibberish, maybe, I don't know. But then she just collapsed, and her body fell back against her bed.

A few others ran in.

I started doing chest compressions, and the patient opened her eyes just a tad bit. She asked faintly, "Is it gone? Is it gone?"

Another nurse told her to relax, that we were going to try to help her.

She shook her head and said, "Tell them I'd never do those things. But I think it's gone now. I feel empty now."

The patient's death was called a few minutes later. The feel in the room was unlike anything I've ever experienced before.

-O.V.
Utah

We once had someone call 911 to report that squirrels kept stealing food from the bird feeder she'd put in her backyard.

A direct quote from this priceless call was, "I already put up 'No Trespassing' signs. Do your jobs and enforce the law. I don't buy bird seed for the squirrels to eat."

I replied, "Ma'am, what do you want me to do? Do you want me to come down there and put the squirrels in cuffs? We can't do that. I don't even know if they make jumpsuits that small."

She cussed, said she was going to call the fire department, and then she hung up on me.

-C.J.

Connecticut

Danger, Danger!

Y'all wouldn't believe the number of submissions I receive detailing wacky reasons why people have called 911 or have called first responders' stations directly. Let's take a look at a few, shall we?

I answered a call at 02:30 from a frantic elderly woman. She said she let her dog out to potty, and that there were 'thousands of frogs' on her patio and in her yard. She was convinced the apocalypse had begun while she was in bed.

I dispatched an officer to her residence. He said there were 'maybe' 10 toads out on the patio, and he assured the caller that she was in no danger. She gave him a baggy filled with dinner mints and thanked him for his service.

-J.S.
Oklahoma

You wouldn't *believe* how many calls we receive through our 911 emergency system *and* our direct line regarding the presidency and/or government happenings lately. We even had someone call 911 to report a Tweet.

-P.I.
New York

We receive calls from angry shoppers ALL. THE. TIME. My favorite was from a woman calling to complain that a popular retailer refused to honor a coupon because it was an e-coupon only, meaning customers could only receive the discount on the item if they ordered online. While I was on the line with the caller, the cashier was on the line with my coworker. Officers arrived and arrested my caller because she had urinated on the merchandise that the cashier refused to discount.

-T.M.

I answered a call from a woman calling to complain that her frozen meal did not contain as many pieces of chicken as the picture on the package showed. I'm an EMT. I don't know what she wanted me to do about it. She cussed me out when I suggested she contact the company to voice her complaints.

-H.T.

Texas

My caller dialed 911 to ask, "Is my neighbor allowed to pull her kids in a wagon?"

Confused, I replied, "I don't see why not. Why would you think it wasn't okay?"

The caller said, "Well, the kids are like four or five. I think it's child abuse because she's stifling their development to walk."

"Does she pull them in the wagon all the time?" I asked.

"Well, no," said the caller. "Maybe like twice a week. But they're old enough to walk. Those kids are gonna grow up and start falling over when they try to use their legs."

-B.R.-D.
Alabama

A caller reported a man in a diner who was 'throwing up gang signs' and 'making a scene' at the counter. She said, "I think he's going to hit the guy or something, so you'd better hurry."

As luck would have it, we had an officer at the place next door, as he'd just stopped for lunch.

The officer had to explain to the caller that the man was deaf and was using sign language to have a discussion with the clerk.

-N.B.
Oregon

We had a pre-teen call our Social Services hotline to report that his father kept logging on the kid's World of Warcraft character and playing the game. The kid wanted his dad to be 'fined or arrested or something.'

A social worker explained that technically, dad was paying for the account. The account was in dad's name.

The kid asked, "Well, can't you tell him he has to make another character or something? He keeps spending all my gold and changing my hearthstone."

No idea what happened with that case.

-T.Y.
New Jersey

A female caller dialed 911 to report a man threatening people with a stick at a school function.

Multiple other callers reported that the original caller was harassing a blind man for using a cane.

When officers arrived on scene, the man stated he did not want the woman to be in trouble; he just wanted her to be educated on disabilities.

-V.W.

South Carolina

I had a woman call to tell me, "Hey, I just bought this new speaker system, and I can't figure out how to turn the volume down. I think my neighbors are gonna start calling you soon. I know it's noisy, but please don't give me a ticket. I've been reading the manual for, like, 20 minutes."

"Okay," I said. "But you might want to call the police department to tell them that."

"That's who I called, right?" she asked.

I laughed and said, "Ma'am, you called a funeral home."

She chuckled and said, "Oh. Well, I guess none of your clients care how loud my music is, huh?"

-N.K.
Florida

---

911 call in the middle of the night to report that the caller's phone went through an OS (operating system) update, and now her Instagram app kept crashing.

When I told her there was nothing I could do about it, she asked, "Don't you have people who can fix this kind of stuff during an emergency?"

"Ma'am," I said, "I hardly think your Instagram app crashing is an emergency."

She told me, "But my friend said my boyfriend commented on his ex's picture, and I have to get a screenshot before he tries to delete it."

I scolded the caller on jamming up the 911 system and warned her that she could face jail time or a fine if she wasted our time on nonsense again.

-G.I.
California

You guys truly have no idea how many people call 911 for cooking directions during holidays. I have documented more than 50 submissions regarding this since I've started this series.

My favorite was from K.L., who said his caller was freaking out because she couldn't make her canned cranberry sauce look like round berries. The dispatcher had to explain to the woman that jellied cranberry sauce wouldn't look that way, and that the caller would have to find a different product.

03:00 911 call for a patient complaining of dry lips.

EMS dispatched. Patient taken by ambulance to ER. ER told patient to buy lip balm.

-C.R.
Georgia

We had a guy call the station one time to report that Wal Mart only had two registers open. He wanted an officer to come out and make a report, so he could include it in his complaint to the store's headquarters.

-R.W.

Iowa

I took a call from a nosy neighbor who wanted the dad across the street arrested for child endangerment. The reason? Dad made his three kids eat their popsicles on the front porch, and the caller complained that 1.) the amount of sugar in the popsicles was a threat to the kids' health, and 2.) the kids' dad was giving them cancer by making them sit under the sun.

The caller complained to us every single day for almost two weeks at the beginning of summer.

We eventually had to enforce our policies on abusing the 911 system. Even after fines, the caller continued to complain and jam our line. The caller was jailed for six days.

911 call to report a 'weird-looking' dog.

I heard someone in the background shout, "Man, what're you doing? Give me that."

Someone snatched the phone out of the caller's hand to explain, "Yo, my guy's never been out in the country before and he's really high right now. It's just an opossum. He's never seen one before. Sorry, man."

We let it slide because the second guy seemed sincere in his apologies. I did, however, tell him he may not want to tell a recorded law enforcement line that he and/or his buddies were participating in drug use.

He said, "Oh damn, you're right. Thanks, man."

-S.X.
New York

I answered a 911 call in the middle of the night from a woman who asked, "If I hand my husband the phone, can you tell him that he *can* get in trouble for peeing in public?"

I heard a man in the background grumble, "I can't get in trouble for pissing off my own porch, Jane. And I wouldn't have to if you didn't spend 20 hours getting ready. But since you have such a huge problem with it, I'll just piss in the kitchen sink next time."

-F.T.
Indiana

I answered a call from a woman who went on a long obscenity-filled tirade because she couldn't find her name on a Coke bottle. She threatened to blow up the gas station.

FYI, that's one of the quickest ways to go to jail.

-A.O.
Location withheld at request

I answered the call from an irate male who stated he was offended by a commercial. The commercial depicted a same-sex couple, and the caller wanted me to ban the television network.

We either have people who think they don't have to listen to us because we don't have power, or we have people who think we have so much power that all we have to do is snap our fingers to change the world.

-C.S.

Georgia

My supervisor was yelling at my partner and me because we may or may not have accidentally backed up into a garbage truck while we were trying to get out of a fast food restaurant parking lot that was located five miles from where we were supposed to be staging.

I tried to lighten the mood by handing my supervisor a Snickers.

She wrote me up.

I can understand the severity of what we did, but I mean, we're medics. I would consider a 'disaster' losing patients, not denting up the rear bumper of an ambulance that's been in service since 1997.

-D.F.
Vermont

I sprained my wrist trying to open a pickle jar after I told my husband, "I can do it, damn." Spent an hour in the waiting room and another hour in the emergency room. I obviously *could not* do it. Gonna be hearing, "I told you so," for the rest of my life.

-G.R.

Oklahoma

Pain in the...

Dispatch received a call from a concerned neighbor who stated she stepped outside to check the mail and could hear screams coming from the house across the street. She stated she did not feel comfortable going to the residence because she did not know her neighbor, and she didn't know what was occurring in the home to make the man scream so loudly. She did not want to walk in on a burglary or a domestic violence situation. She also told dispatch that the man had company 'all hours of the day and night,' so she suspected he was involved with drugs. EMS and two of our guys (my partner and I) arrived on scene.

We told EMS to hang back while we approached the front porch. Indeed, there was a great deal of screaming coming from inside the residence. A male sounded like he was in pain, and he shouted for help every few seconds.

My partner knocked loudly on the front door, and then we heard, "Help me! Come upstairs and help me!"

The front door was unlocked, so we let ourselves in and cautiously made our way to the attic.

I stopped in the doorway and just stared at the man.

My partner exclaimed, "What the hell?"

The resident was naked, and he was hanging by one ankle (connected by a thick rope) to a beam in the ceiling. It appeared his other ankle had been tied as well, but that rope had broken. There was a plastic chair nearby, tipped over.

I didn't mean to ask aloud, but the words slipped out.

"Is this some kind of weird sex thing?" I asked.

"What?" the man asked. "No! Get me down. It hurts so bad."

I held the man's upper body, while my partner stood on the plastic chair and used his multi-tool to cut the rope. Gravity got the best of us, and I dropped the man. He whacked his head on the floor good and started cussing.

"What the hell were you doing up there?" my partner asked.

"My back hurt," the man said.

"So you got naked and hung yourself from the ceiling?" I asked in an inadvertent incredulous tone.

The man said that he'd seen something online that said hanging upside down could stretch and realign the spine. He stated that he couldn't afford the gadget he'd seen advertised, and he couldn't afford an inversion table, so he got the bright idea to tie his ankles to a beam in the attic. He failed to think ahead on how he would get down. He told us that he tried to 'do a crunch' and reach the rope, but he did not have the physical strength to do that.

"Okay," I said. "But why are you naked?"

He countered, "Do I need to have a reason for being naked in my own house?"

"Fair enough," I replied.

The patient's ankle was swollen and bruised. We called EMS inside, and they commented that the man's ankle looked broken. They took him to the hospital and when we caught up again, they said the ER told them later that the man had broken his ankle.

I guess the resident told EMS that he'd been hanging upside down for nearly an hour, and he had to keep swinging and attempting to pull himself up to prevent losing consciousness.

When my partner and I left the residence, the neighbor across the street flagged us down. We told her that we could not discuss the details of our run, but that the case did not appear to involve drugs or violence. She seemed relieved.

-P.G.
Wisconsin

I worked with a guy who was fired about a week after he got hired on. A coworker caught the guy using our birthing simulator as a sex toy. He didn't even pull his pants up when he was caught. He just finished what he was doing like it was no big deal.

*A birthing simulator is a device shaped like a pregnant belly and oftentimes upper thighs. It usually includes a 'baby' that comes out of a vaginal opening. This device is used to teach different birthing scenarios.

-R.W.
South Carolina

Jumping to Conclusions

A call came over the radio reporting a possible B&E at an apartment complex. Nobody jumped at the chance to respond, so I headed that way.

When I arrived on scene, I spotted a potential subject. He stuck out like a blind carpenter's thumb, as he was the only person in the hallway with a wobbly tower of DVDs stacked on top of the two gaming consoles he struggled to carry. He appeared nervous and kept scanning his surroundings. I knew he was my guy when he spotted me, dropped everything, and sprinted back into the apartment that he'd just exited.

I chased the subject through the apartment and out onto the balcony. Surely, I thought, he would realize that we were four stories up, and he would surrender. It wasn't like there was anywhere for him to go, right?

The subject attempted to leap from the balcony on which we were standing to a balcony attached to the neighboring building. The gap between the buildings was probably about five to six feet wide.

I think my exact words as I realized he was about to make the jump were, "No, no, no, no!"

How stupid I was to think I could even stop him.

For a split second, I thought the subject was going to make a clean getaway. He managed to grab the awning of the neighboring balcony, and he had one leg over the iron wrought fencing. When he tried to put down his other foot, though, he slipped. The subject plummeted approximately 40 feet, and the atmosphere erupted with deafening screams from below. I was too afraid to even look down.

When I finally convinced myself to take a peek, I was awfully surprised. The subject was not a splattered mess. He had flattened a couple of bushes, but otherwise appeared in decent shape. Thankfully, he was too out of it to run again, so I stood over him while we awaited the arrival of EMS.

When I explained that he was under arrest for his burglary antics, he appeared dazed and confused.

"How can I rob my own apartment?" he asked.

"Your apartment? That was your apartment?"

He winced as he nodded and said, "Yeah. I live there."

"If you live there," I said with a huff, "then why did you drop everything and run when you saw me?"

He groaned and said, "Because I just broke up with my girl and thought she called you all 'cause I just bought weed."

I shook my head in amazement and asked, "Then what were you doing with all that stuff?"

He responded, "She won't give her key back, so I'm taking all my stuff over to my brother's place. That way, she can't take it and sell it on Craigslist."

His story checked out. He was not in possession of marijuana or paraphernalia, nor did he really do anything wrong. I realized during his medical transport that I never actually ordered him to stop, so I guess I can understand from his point of view why it was so frightening to see me. Thankfully, he accepted my apology and I his, and we chalked the incident up to jumping to conclusions.

I found out later that the B&E that was called in from the fourth floor was another case of mistaken identity, so no apartments had been burglarized that afternoon. My subject's neighbor witnessed the whole ordeal and took the DVDs and gaming consoles inside for safe keeping.

The subject, miraculously, only came out with a few scratches and complained of being sore.

-L.J.
Florida

You've Goat to be Kidding Me

My supervisor demanded to know how I became so distracted that I veered off the road and uprooted a telephone pole from the ground.

My partner and I explained that we did not expect our patient to come barreling across the street one block from the residence reported by dispatch, *completely nude*, carrying a pygmy goat (who wearing a sweater and had pool noodles over its horns) over his shoulders.

I mean, come on. You see something like that, you're gonna get distracted, right?

We watched an LEO roll up, tase the subject (which did absolutely *nothing*), wrestle him to the ground (a bystander saved the goat from walking into oncoming traffic— imagine telling that story to your friends), and then we put an end to it with a big ole' dose of ketamine.

We had to wait for a tow truck and an additional unit for patient transport, but we got to play with a goat until Animal Control arrived, so that was cool.

I still have *no freaking idea* what transpired before all that went down, so I'm just as confused as you are.

-S.S.
Ohio

I've been lucky enough to say that my horse has only been assaulted in the line of duty once—and only once.

A drunk passerby thought it would be funny to run towards us at full speed and punch my horse in her mouth.

My horse, trained to remain calm in any situation, wasn't having any part of it. She promptly whipped around and returned the gesture by kicking the subject in *his* mouth.

Night in jail, community service, hefty fines, and whatever it cost the guy to get an implant where his tooth had been.

-J.E.

Louisiana

New Year, Same Old Me

First responders share some of their calls from past New Year's Eve/New Year's Day, and the days surrounding the two. I don't know how you do it, guys!

We responded to a single vehicle accident, after the car had run into a steep drainage ditch. According to the designated driver, one of the drunk passengers in the backseat set off a cluster of bottle rockets inside the vehicle. Everyone except the firework-happy passenger declined medical treatment. Some of the patient's injuries were sustained from the fireworks, while most appeared to have been sustained from the designated driver beating the ever-living crap out of the patient.

-Initials and location withheld at request

"2018 is gonna be my year," I said to my coworkers. "My first patient of the year is going to set the tone for the rest of my year."

I said this about 20 seconds before Charge assigned the patient presenting at midnight to the ER for a pregnancy test. And yes, she was accompanied by about 10 friends who were already planning her baby shower. She wasn't pregnant.

I kept track, first as a joke but then because it started getting ridiculous. This year alone, I (not counting my shift coworkers or our department as a whole) have been assigned to 207 patients seeking pregnancy tests.

This year I said, "2019 is gonna be my year. Quick, someone give me a winning lottery ticket."

-K.E.
California

---

911 call from a concerned neighbor who witnessed the guy across the street doing something incredibly dangerous and stupid.

She said she tried to talk him out of it, but he just wouldn't listen. She wanted an officer to swing by his house and try to talk some sense into him.

I was that officer, and yeah, I have no idea what the guy was thinking. He duct-taped three metal ladders together, and I found him trying to knock a boot off a live wire by extending a broom up there.

He insisted he was *not* suicidal, just really drunk and wanting his shoe back after 'accidentally' throwing it over the line.

-H.M.

Tennessee

I stopped a motorist on his way home. He was operating a motorcycle while under the influence of alcohol. His passenger was a plastic 4-ft-tall Virgin Mary decoration he'd swiped from someone's Nativity scene. He said he couldn't find his helmet, so he was wearing a bucket with holes cut out for his eyes.

I have no idea how he managed to get as far as he did because he couldn't even stand on his own for more than a few seconds.

-P.U.

Florida (Author's Note: FLORIDA!)

Our station either transported or treated on site six cases involving patients being shot in the eye with corks from alcohol bottles.

-D.L.

Nevada

House party with 40+ drunken attendees. Someone decided it would be a good idea to ride a bicycle off the roof. But don't worry, he prepared! Dude tied a fitted sheet around his neck, so it would catch wind and act like a parachute. (It didn't, by the way.)

What concerns me most is that nobody claimed to have talked him out of it. Then again, if someone tells me they're going to do something stupid, I usually give a sly smile and say, "You should do that." Not because it's a good idea, but because I know I'm about to benefit from that person's stupidity. That probably makes me a bad person, but oh well.

Riding a bicycle off the roof of a huge Victorian house went about as good as you can imagine it would.

Thankfully, the patient only appeared to have a few broken bones.

The *greatest* thing about this is that the patient already had a cast on one of his extremities, so he apparently has a history of doing stupid effing things.

I won't even tell you what his BAC turned out to be, but aim high.

-S.T.-W.
Missouri

It was 10-degrees outside, and I was on a team designated to dismantle a plastic slide at a local playground…at 02:00.

Our highly intoxicated patient, for some odd reason, tried to climb the slide from the bottom up, slipped, and somehow became lodged in the tube. Her friends called 911 after an *hour*.

We (fire department) assisted, while a few guys from the PD stood by for 'emotional support.' The patient was covered in vomit and had urinated on herself. She was unconscious when we finally managed to pull her out. EMS transported her to the hospital.

All subjects on site were underage, so they were taken in by the cops.

-L.D.

North Dakota

We were dispatched alongside the FD because an elderly caller complained that she could smell gas when she woke up in the dead of night to get a glass of water from the kitchen. Upon arrival, we could also smell gas.

Two guys from the fire department were able to figure out that the dial on the caller's stove was turned just enough to emit gas into the kitchen.

The caller cussed and said her cat had been getting up on the stove lately. She believed the cat must have accidentally turned the dial this time.

We helped the caller air out her residence and she talked with my partner until she felt safe enough to go inside. We suggested she use a water bottle or crinkled aluminum foil placed across the stovetop to teach the cat to stay down.

-F.E.

Montana

Rough Day

I stood up too quickly, became dizzy, and fell face-first into my glass coffee table. There was blood *everywhere*. Because I really don't live too far from the nearest hospital, I put a towel down on my driver's seat and drove myself.

I was pleasantly surprised to see the emergency room offered a valet service. Since I was still bleeding, I took advantage of this service.

When I went inside, one of the male clerks turned white, ran away, and returned with a nurse. She made me sit in a wheelchair, and she took me straight back.

I have read all your books. I don't work in the healthcare field. There I was, thinking that my injuries were 'not that bad,' but all the ER staff I encountered gasped or would exclaim, "Oh my!" That left me with a pit in my stomach because when the people in your books say that, it's usually not a good sign.

About 15 minutes later, while these nurses were using tweezers to pick out shards of glass from my face, someone knocked on the door.

I glanced up and saw one of the men from the valet service. He was red in the face. I thought he was going to tell me that he wrecked my pride and joy, a vintage sports car that I had recently restored.

Instead, he said to me, "I'm sorry to bother you, but do you think you could come move your car?"

I was baffled and angry. I grumbled, "Well, what's the damn point of having valet service in the first place?"

I then went on a rant about young people and their work ethics because I really didn't think it through. I was in pain, was embarrassed about my condition, and despite having decent insurance, all I could think about was the hospital bill.

The guy shook his head and said, "It's not that. Sir, we can't find anyone who knows how to drive a manual."

With strips of gauze hanging off portions of my face, and with blood still gushing out of my wounds, I exited the emergency room and parked my vehicle. I wasn't even angry at this point. In fact, I was thankful the young men came to get me, rather than *trying* to drive my car. I would have really been heated if someone had burned out my clutch.

As I went back to my room to get patched up, other patients waiting to be seen or admitted were jumping out of my way like I had the plague or something. I caught a glimpse of myself in the security mirror hanging from the corner, and I looked like Frankenstein's monster.

After a good chunk of time spent in the emergency room, I was discharged with 37 sutures, two areas that had been glued shut, and a swollen, mangled face. The doctor wrote up a prescription for three days' worth of pain pills, and I really appreciated that gesture because I was not feeling my best upon being discharged.

That's actually not even the worst part. I had never even thought to call my wife at work to let her know what I'd gotten myself into, so she and I arrived home around the same time. She was irate, but mostly because I didn't tell her I had gone to the emergency room.

It took another three hours to get the glass fully cleaned up and scrub the blood trail out of the carpets. My wife was also upset because I bled on a (ONE) stupid throw pillow, but I'm not sure why because she only has 40 more of the damn things around the house.

-J.Y.
California

Hairy Situation

Back in the early-80s, when I hadn't a clue what to do with my life, I'd seen a local ad for paramedic training. I had missed all the college cutoff dates and was going nowhere in life, so I thought, 'Why not?'

It turned out that I enjoyed the classes. I liked the rush of arriving on scene and never knowing what to expect. I felt purpose for the first time in my life. I liked having to think on my feet. I eventually became certified and was released to the hounds.

I'll never forget my first shift as a real, live medic. The feel of the day was already different because I was *legitimate* now. I wasn't just some peon anymore. Admittedly, I was a bit full of myself, but I think I was just proud that I could say I was doing something with my life now.

Anyway, we were dispatched to a local shopping center. It was rather busy, it being a holiday weekend. I could hear nothing but murmurs and screams as I entered the building with my partner following behind me.

A crowd had gathered at the escalators. Both sides were packed with people. Neither side was moving. It didn't click in my head yet. I still didn't know what to expect. Dispatch hadn't told us too much.

As soon as I saw the patient, I turned around and vomited. I was so embarrassed. I had ralphed up my lunch in front of close to 50 bystanders. Nobody seemed to notice, though, because they were all focused on the patient.

The female patient was lying on the ground, partially scalped. Most of her hair was still caught up in the escalator gears. One section of her hair that hadn't caught reached down to her ankles. She was in a state of shock and I don't think she could have stopped screaming even if she'd wanted to.

I have no idea how this patient was not in worse condition. Bystanders stated that a security guard had noticed the patient struggling after stepping off the escalator, but by the time the guard had managed to shut the system down, it was simply too late. Others had rushed to her aide and attempted to pull her hair out from the gears, but they couldn't. Two men told the woman to lie down.

We had to cut the patient's hair in order to transport her. To give you an idea of how bad this was, I think we cut to about the middle of her neck or just below. And, like I said, the rest of her hair had been down to her ankles. I still have no idea how the escalator didn't jam up. It had been intermittently smoking while we were on scene, however, so I'm sure it was at its breaking point.

The patient was transported by air to a larger facility, and to this day, I still have no idea what became of her. I would imagine that she underwent multiple surgeries and had a long road to recovery. I can also only assume that she needed some sort of emotional therapy for the incident.

I hadn't really given the incident much thought over the years, but the other day, a new medic joined our station. She vomited on scene and began crying because she was so embarrassed by her reaction to trauma. It just brought back so many memories, including this one, that I thought I'd forgotten.

Thinking about it now, after all these years, I still feel ill. I think it must be more emotional than physical, because I have seen much more gruesome injuries since then.

I have been an 'escalator warrior' since the incident, so if I'm out and about and see someone with a dragging shoelace, purse strap, or other accessory or whatnot, I'll speak up and tell them, "You might want to fix that before you get caught up." Most of the time, people look at me like I'm insane. But, because of what I witnessed, I don't feel too bad about warning others.

-Initials and location withheld at request

We responded to a fire at a grocery store and someone had illegally parked in the striped lane with message 'FIRE LANE ONLY, DO NOT PARK' painted on the asphalt, directly in front of the hydrant and where a fire truck needed to be.

I watched the driver of the firetruck ram right into the tiny sedan until he could get it pushed out of the way. He hit it so hard on the third ram that the bumper fell off.

Not sure what happened with that, really, since I was new to EMS and the driver was a volunteer with the FD. I'm not saying he was *right* in doing that, but it's always stuck in my mind.

-R.S.

Virginia

Damn, What Kind of Pie Was It?

I wasn't having the best day, and all my coworkers knew. My boyfriend told me at 05:30 that he'd been cheating on me and wanted to 'explore his options.' I cried a little bit, but then I told him I had to go to work. I didn't yell or break anything or fight with him. I simply continued with my morning routine the best I could, and I left for work. I tried not to let it get to me, but my nerves were shot. I ended up spilling a latte all over myself while I was in the car. I cried and cried because of that and my relationship drama, so my eyes were swollen. Traffic was horrendous, so I was late for work. I was written up for being late and 'being a mess.' One of the nurses let me use a pair of her scrub pants that didn't look so much like scrubs, so at least that was a plus.

The shift started off with a bang, and I mean that regarding a patient. The guy had accidentally dropped his gun and shot himself in the thigh…in a mall bathroom. He wasn't a very nice person, and I left his room in tears. Ordinarily, I have thick skin, but I couldn't handle anything else, and I'd only been at work 30 minutes.

Throughout the day, patients flooded in for even more pressing issues. I know, I know, you're probably thinking, 'What could be more pressing than a GSW?' Well, let's see. I think we had four codes in the span of an hour. We had quite a few ODs. We had several MVAs. Throw in a few stemis for good measure. It was nonstop.

With an hour left to go, I noticed a frequent flyer approaching the building. My coworker saw her first, though, and took off, leaving me the one to deal with the woman's abrasive behavior. Nobody liked this patient. She was rude, crude, and even if she came in with a papercut to her finger, she believed she had all the right in the world to be treated first. What's worse is that she was an active drug seeker, and when she didn't get her way (either being seen first, getting drugs, or getting what she wanted in general), she became violent. She had been trespassed from the grounds already, but the law requires that if a patient presents with a medical need, we have to register them.

Jane walked to the desk just fine.

"Get me a doctor," she demanded.

"What's going on today, Miss Doe?"

"Just get me a doctor," she shouted at me, cursing along the way.

I sighed and said, "You know I can't do that unless you tell me what's wrong."

She told me, "My legs hurt. I can't walk."

I didn't argue with her because 1.) that's not my job, 2.) you can't argue with stupid, and 3.) I really wasn't in the mood.

I registered Jane, watched her pop up on my tracking board, and I told her someone would see her when it was her turn.

Of course, she started shouting at me and slamming her fists on my counter.

I lost my temper and told her, "If you don't go sit down right now, I'm calling the cops. I'm not even calling security this time because I'm sick of you coming in here and treating everyone like shit."

Jane threw herself on the ground and started screaming about medical neglect. Other patients were coming and going left and right, and some of them looked at me like I was Satan because I wasn't rushing out to the lobby to help this older woman get off the floor. Some patients tried to help Jane into a wheelchair, but she refused. She just wanted to roll around on the floor and throw a temper tantrum until someone got fed up with her behavior and called her back, just so we could see her and discharge her.

I told Jane that she could kick and scream all she wanted, and that I didn't care this time. Triage came for another patient and ended up calling security because she saw I had just continued about my day and was ignoring Jane's behavior. The nurse didn't scold me or anything. I think she was secretly on my side.

Jane started dragging herself around the lobby like that half-body zombie in the first episode of *The Walking Dead*. She was using her arms and upper body strength to drag herself around the lobby, and she just couldn't be quiet while she was doing it.

Security arrived, and they were trying to get Jane off the floor. She started screaming more and louder. When a guard touched her arm (touched, not grabbed), Jane started shouting about police brutality and began begging bystanders to record the incident for her attorney's use.

People were buying into this. I think the better term would be, they were eating it up like candy. Everyone wanted to be a part of the drama, so we had two or three bystanders recording the incident. They were even telling security, "Come on, leave her alone. She's hurt, man."

A bystander even came up to me to say, "What you're doing to that patient is wrong. She really deserves to be treated before all these people that you're calling back. Shame on you."

Before I even had a chance to respond, an administrator came over the PA system and announced, "It's Patient Appreciation Day. Come down to the cafeteria for free pie and ice cream. Sugar-free desserts and fruit are also available. Everything is free!"

I kid you not, Jane became a CrossFit expert or something because she leapt up off the floor using only the strength of her lower body. She seriously *jumped* up like I see people doing at the gym. I work out a few times a week and I'm not even sure that I have the strength to do what she did.

I dryly thought to myself, 'It's a miracle. Jane is cured.'

The bystander who'd come to complain kind of looked at Jane, then looked at me, then looked at Jane again. He/she then said, "I get it. Sorry for yelling at you."

I just kind of smiled like, 'Yeah, told you so,' even though I hadn't said a thing.

One of the guards asked, "Do you still want to be seen?"

I shot him a look that could kill.

Jane waved him off and said, "Yeah, yeah. I'll come back after I get my free pie."

Jane high-tailed it down to the cafeteria for her cure-all pie, so when Triage called her name a few minutes later, she wasn't around. We marked her as LBT.

I went home for the day, and my boyfriend met me in the driveway with flowers and a ring. He told me he wanted to see how I would react if he 'told me the worst,' and then he asked me to marry him. I told him no, and I told him to move out. That's seriously how fed up I was with everyone's crap.

My coworker texted me at the end of her shift and told me that Jane had come back to be seen. Charge made her wait longer because she had been an LBT earlier. I guess Jane tried to headbutt the security glass on our department door, but she couldn't break through it. I guess the cops were called, but I've seen Jane since then and nothing's really changed. Kind of wish we'd have more 'free pie days' in the cafeteria so she'd leave us alone.

-J.P.

Indiana

True freaking story:

Instead of calling 911, a man chained an office chair to his riding lawnmower and pulled his wife to our ER.

He was arrested for DUI, and his wife was later arrested for possession.

-F.I.

Location withheld at request

A.F. sent in this submission on behalf of her retired RN great-grandmother, E.B., whom she reads the series to as part of a technique to assist with Alzheimer's.

Many years ago, one of my coworkers was fired for performing sexual acts on residents. She was in her teens, receiving monetary bribes to perform sexual acts on/with residents who were 65+.

She and I graduated from the same nursing program, and I considered her one of my best friends.

She was caught when a candy striper entered the room. I believe she was stripped of her certification.

We were all more conservative back then, so I ended our friendship because I was afraid to be linked with that sort of behavior.

<u>Christmas Spirit</u>

I work at a large hospital on Orthopedics, but this submission did not take place at my workplace. After reading your books, I must admit that I have gained an appreciation for my 'boring' job.

My mother recently moved in with us. We rarely decorate for holidays, and even when we do, it's usually nothing more than a festive wreath on the front door. My mother, however, found this 'just plain wrong,' so she went all out this year. It was annoying at first, but we opened up to the idea of having a fully decorated home.

My mother put garland on our staircase, jingle bells on doorknobs, and even replaced our old Domino's Pizza magnets with magnets shaped like reindeer. Outside, she *really* went wild. Our front yard looked like the North Pole. We had inflatable decorations, plastic reindeer 'taking off' with Santa's sleigh, had huge plastic candy canes lining our walkway…It was beautiful, honestly.

Our front porch was also filled with decorations. My mother put snow globes all along the railings, put up five strands of lights, changed the globe on our front porch light to look like a snowman's head, and she sprayed our windows with fake snow. Her pride and joy, however, was this gigantic five-foot-something animatronic Santa she'd found at a yard sale for $10. I bet the thing would have cost hundreds of dollars brand-new. It had some kind of motion detector in it, so if you walked by the house at just the right angle, it would rotate, wave, wish you a Merry Christmas, and then sing.

We were finishing up with supper that night, when we heard commotion out front. My husband was working late, and I wasn't about to send my teenage son outside, so I cautiously opened the front door (I couldn't see out because of the fake snow—thanks to my mother) just in time to see a man pull his shirt off and toss it to the ground. He then *attacked* the Santa decoration and body slammed it to the ground!

I should have closed and locked the door right away, but I was so infuriated that instead, I ran out on the porch and screamed, "Stop! What are you doing?"

I could tell right away that the man was either stoned or drunk. He shouted at me to mind my own business, and then he started punching the Santa decoration while it was on the ground. The man had damaged the speaker inside, so the decoration's Merry Christmas message was coming out all garbled.

The man screamed, "You don't get to tell people how to feel!"

By this point, my mother had dialed 911, and two officers came out. They tried to arrest the man without using force, but his behavior was erratic and violent. He grabbed a metal stake that was tying down one side of an inflatable decoration, so as soon as he yanked that up from the ground, our decoration toppled. The officers had to tase the man in my front yard, while my son watched from his bedroom window, I stood near my front door, and my mother stood behind me. She was in tears over this, but not because the man had essentially ruined all her hard work, but because she felt saddened by his condition.

One of the officers explained to me that the patient appeared to be under the influence of crystal meth, which would certainly explain away a lot of his behavior.

It was too close to Christmas to bother replacing the damaged decorations, so I promised my mother we would buy new, better decorations for next Christmas.

-S.G.

Maine

"Oh, he's just playing!" said the intoxicated man who was trying to climb through my kitchen window as my 115-pound Rott-Pin mix snarled and barked.

I must have told the man a thousand times to drop the knife he had in his hand, do not enter my house, and do not approach me, but did he listen?

My dog bit as soon as the man got within three feet of me and held him until cops could arrive. Dispatch had to replace my husband on a last-minute heart Cath transport call because I thought I went into premature labor from all the stress.

I was fine, the baby was fine, my husband was fine, and my dog got a steak for dinner. The intruder got something like three stitches and a long time in county jail.

-M.S.
Georgia

The Plan

We were messing around at the station one day, when our football got kicked up on the roof. We couldn't figure out a way to get up there because the top level was locked, so we grabbed a ladder from the supply closet. The plan was I would stand on the ladder, and my coworkers would lift it in the air, so that I could reach the gutter and pull myself up on the roof.

They lifted the ladder, but it started wobbling as I was reaching for the gutter. I tried to make a hop for it, but I missed the gutter, fell off the ladder, and basically scraped my face down the side of the brick building before I landed on my already-bad knee.

A female coworker walked by and said, "You do know there's a ladder attached to the back part of the building that leads to a fire escape, right?"

Well no, we did not know that, or we would have just done it that way.

One of my male coworkers looked me dead in the eyes and said, "Bro, I think this is why women live longer than men."

I think he could be right.

-M.I.
South Dakota

<u>Arts and... Crap I'm Tired</u>

My wife paints and stains wooden signs and sells them on Etsy. I cut the boards for her and for items such decorative birdhouses, I cut and assemble them.

After a 48-hour shift and getting virtually no sleep during that time or the 30 hours prior to that shift, I decided to hurry through assembling some of my wife's merchandise. That way, I could get all the sleep I needed, and she could keep busy with work.

Well, I was so tired that I wasn't thinking clearly. I sat down at my workbench, but for some reason my brain didn't think to use the clamps I have. I placed two boards on my lap and was going to use the nail gun to drive them together.

Yeah, you guessed it. The nail went through both boards and into my thigh. I was bleeding profusely and passed out from a combination of shock and exhaustion.

My wife had heard the thud of me going down and taking half of my workstation with me. She placed a call to the station, and some of my off-the-clock coworkers came over and patched me up. It's not something we probably *should* have done, but there was no sense in paying thousands of dollars for a doctor to pull a nail out of my leg, clean me up, and slap a bandage over the wound.

It took a while to heal, but the wound *did* heal.

Rest assured, I will not be using the nail gun or any other power tool unless I get at least three hours of sleep before I need to use it/them.

-G.H.
Colorado

<u>Best Laid Plans</u>

A lot of people seem to think that because I am a firefighter, I *only* respond to calls regarding fires. This is simply not true. I work with search and rescue, perform on-scene vehicle extractions, and I perform emergency intervention treatment such as stabilizing a patient or performing CPR if I am on scene before a medic.

Not long ago, we received a complaint of a crushed vehicle at a rural business. We weren't sure what to expect because the caller was an elderly woman who couldn't give us much information. She said a tractor had been involved.

We notified EMS and the PD before we headed that way. Unfortunately, because we didn't know what was going on, we didn't have a lot to report to the other departments. They were sort of irritated with us, but eh, what can you do, am I right?

On scene, the guys and I were just too dumbfounded to say much of anything. We

213

were going to have to perform an extraction. That much was clear.

A small pickup truck from the early 1990s was parked directly under the second-story window (more like a glass garage door) of this tractor supply store. The truck was crushed, and the driver was stuck in a leaning position from the driver's side to the passenger seat. There was an expensive riding lawnmower on top of the pickup.

The owner of the shop explained that the customer wanted to purchase the mower. However, the mower was near the front of the building, and there were several mowers behind it. It would have taken 'a really long time' to move the other mowers and drive this mower down the ramp and out the lower exit. So, the customer and the store owner decided they would open the window, tie a few canvas straps to the mower, and a bunch of guys would slowly lower it into the bed of the customer's pickup.

As you've probably deduced, the guys couldn't support the weight of the mower and the customer had not pulled up enough, so everyone involved pretty much dropped this

$6,000 zero-turn mower out the window, crushed the customer's truck, ruined the mower, and trapped the customer in his vehicle.

It took about 20 minutes to get the guy out of his truck. He had a few bruises and scrapes, but he was fine otherwise.

No idea who was going to pay for what. My job was done, so the guys and I went back to the station.

-C.R.

Iowa

Undercover

In the early 90s, I was part of a unit that conducted undercover investigations and stings. I was most commonly involved with illegal drug activity, mainly cocaine and heroin.

Once I made the deal with the suspect in question, he rounded the corner and was met by my coworkers.

This man retrieved identification from his pocket and told my coworkers that he was also an officer.

In addition to a drug charge, he was charged with impersonating an officer. He swore up and down that he was not involved with the assault that occurred for the suspect to gain access to the identification, but he volunteered this information prior to our guys mentioning that fact. He backtracked and incriminated himself…not just for the assault, but also naming himself as the suspect responsible for robbing a liquor store at gunpoint (that resulted in a murder), and several other charges.

I don't know if he was the dumbest person in the world for thinking that he could make us believe he was an officer, or if he was the dumbest person in the world for ratting himself out for the rest of his crimes.

He went away for a *long* time.

-Initials and location withheld at request

The $20,000 Cruiser

Way back when, our department received a new cruiser. A new $20,000 cruiser. New $20,000 cruiser that didn't even have 100 miles on it yet.

I was assigned the $20,000 cruiser, and I loved it. Everyone else jokingly (or partially jokingly) hated me for it.

I had just responded to a domestic at a home in the country, so I was headed back to town, flying down a rural road at approximately 55 MPH.

I'm still not sure how this happened, but before I knew it, a whooping crane flew right through the open passenger window, obstructed my vision of the roadway, and this resulted in me crashing a new $20,000 cruiser.

The bird couldn't manage to get itself out of my car, so as soon as I realized I was okay (saved by the airbag and my seatbelt), I called for backup and *left the bird* in my cruiser until someone could confirm my account. I didn't think anyone was going to believe me.

DNR (Department of Natural Resources) came out and measured this bird as standing about 4 ½ feet tall, with a wingspan of just over 6 feet. They took the bird in for a wing injury. A 16.4-pound bird basically totaled a $20,000 cruiser.

I keep reiterating the price of this car because this is all I heard for six months straight. **Everyone** gave me crap about it.

If I mentioned grabbing a coffee I'd hear, "Yeah, gotta be alert so you don't wreck another $20,000 car."

If I mentioned my day off, someone would say, "You already crashed a $20,000 cruiser. Don't go crashing your truck."

We eventually replaced my cruiser and received a few more…which made my coworkers pester me even more. All I heard all year long was, "Hey, we just got these cruisers. Don't pull a John and wreck one."

-R.G.
Illinois

We arrested two females in their late teens. They were booked for disorderly conduct, public intoxication, and battery.

I think it took about five minutes to get a mugshot from each female because we had to keep saying, "Stop making the duck lips, please. Look at the camera, please. No, you can't make the peace sign. No, we're not going to stand on a chair to get a better angle. No, we do not edit the pictures."

We finally just settled on a random shot. One female was crying because we were 'being really mean,' and the other had her eyes closed.

I doubt they have much to worry about. Their friends probably won't be able to recognize them without their animal-ear filters, anyway.

-O.C.
New Jersey

<u>Craving Freedom</u>

I do my best not to be judgmental, but there are times I just have to shake my head. When I responded to a call of a shoplifter, I didn't have a pregnant woman pictured as the suspect. I could understand if the suspect had been caught stealing food, baby items, or personal hygiene supplies, but she'd been caught by staff and on film for stealing batteries, magazines, lipstick, and other non-essential items. She wasn't homeless. She wasn't a stereotype. She was a spoiled brat from a nice family, who lived in a nice house (which we learned her parents had purchased for her), drove a $60,000 SUV, and had everything a person could ask for, if you ask me.

The suspect was already outside the store when I pulled up. Once she saw me, she took off running. She was about six months pregnant, and I honestly don't know how she moved as quickly as she did. I certainly was not going to be the one to deploy a taser on a

221

pregnant suspect, so I called for backup, got in my patrol, and followed the suspect until she ran out of breath.

I learned the suspect had warrants for theft and such, so she was processed into our facility. It appeared she enjoyed participating in crimes for the thrill. She was sentenced to our jail for 30 days, which was considered a light sentence for the charges. She did have a prenatal examination, and she was scheduled for a wellness check weekly, just as part as our facility's procedures.

This woman was the worst inmate ever, and just because she was annoying and temperamental. Sure, I bet some of that happened to be hormones. But most of it was not. She felt entitled, and I didn't know how else to explain it to her than, "You. Are. In. Jail." I told her we weren't running a resort when she would demand a hot bath or a back massage. She used her visitation time and calls to complain to her parents and sister that we were 'abusing' her. Her parents threatened us with a lawsuit when we told them they could not bring food to the woman.

We just shrugged and handed them a guidebook that contained our facility policies.

One night, this woman threw a huge fit because she said she was craving Taco Bell, and she wanted us to go get food for her. We have done that *once* for an inmate, and it was only because he had a cognitive disability and was in jail on a technicality. None of us believed he should have been locked up in the first place, so yes, he received special treatment. I don't even think he was ever even in a cell. As I recall it, he spent most of his time sitting in an administrator's office, watching TV and looking at the pictures in magazines.

We explained to the pregnant inmate that we could not and would not fetch her fast food, and sorry, but that's something everyone should consider before going out and committing a crime.

This woman had a complete meltdown. She tore her clothes off and started punching herself in the stomach, stating if we didn't go get her Taco Bell, she would kill her baby.

We transported her to the hospital for treatment and felt she needed a psych eval as well. Two officers accompanied her to the ER. She spoke to a counselor and told them that we had been mistreating her.

Boy, things got messy real quick. The patient told the counselor that if she went back to jail, she would 'find a way' to commit suicide, but first she would find a way to terminate her pregnancy. She said she 'wasn't crazy' and she had no history of mental instability of which we were aware (I'm not sure we would be privy to that information, anyhow). She said that she was tired of being controlled by us, and she said, "I'm tired of hearing 'No, no, no' every damn time I tell them I want something. I pay your salary with my taxes, so you work for me."

I know it sounds like a case of temporary insanity or maybe it sounds like the woman was off her meds or something, but I can squash those suspicions because the woman flat-out told officers, nurses, and even the counselor that she was tired of being locked up, and she would do and say 'anything necessary' to make us let her out. She stated she knew her best chance to get us to do what she wanted was to threaten to harm herself or the baby because, "Then you will get in trouble for letting me do anything while I'm in custody." She complained some more about being locked up and not being able to do what she wanted. Basically, we had to tell her, "Tough titty."

The counselor suggested the ER keep her for a little bit as a 'reset,' hoping that spending some time out of jail would allow her to 'refresh' and 'adjust her attitude.' That was fine with us. We kept officers posted outside her room.

The patient pressed her call button 19 times in 30 minutes and assaulted two nurses because they refused to order her pizza.

Back to jail.

We kept her on suicide watch, which took away even more of her freedom, which made her scream and scream and scream. She became hoarse and I swear, some of our other long-term inmates began clapping once they realized she couldn't scream anymore.

I think we went through a meltdown regarding her cravings at least twice a day for 30 days. She seemed to be under the impression that when you're in jail, you still get what you want. Hell, even when she was not in jail, she apparently felt she could do what she wanted, when she wanted, with zero repercussions. It doesn't quite work that way.

-Initials and location withheld at request

As with most places nowadays, our mugshots are subject to internet placement. That means if you're arrested and have your picture taken, it's gonna show up online with your charges placed underneath your picture.

I have personally answered no fewer than 10 calls from subjects regarding these mugshots. Only two have wanted them removed. The others wanted a chance to take the pictures again because they said the mugshot was a bad shot, bad angle, or had bad lighting.

Just don't get arrested in the first place, and you won't have to worry about looking like crap for the whole world to see! That's my advice, anyway.

J.C.
Vermont

What Did You Think Would Happen?!

Healthcare workers and LEOs share some (more) stupid things their patients and subjects have done. What in the world are people thinking?

We transferred a patient out via helicopter after he'd come to us in nasty shape. His friends said he'd gotten drunk, grabbed a raccoon, and tried to kiss it. When the love connection failed, the patient tripped and landed on top of a bonfire.

The patient was missing a portion of his upper lip, had corneal scratches, needed sutures to multiple facial lacerations, and sustained severe burns to his face, arms, and chest.

-K.I.
Ohio

I had to let my partner deal with a patient who'd rubbed Vaseline on his penis and lit it on fire.

The only thing he said to us while he was conscious was, "The internet said it wasn't going to burn."

Buddy, the internet lied to you.

-V.A.

West Virginia

If you're going to cause a scene that requires police presence, try to use that little brain of yours so we can just arrest you and leave, rather than making it an hour-long circus.

Our guy was angry that his neighbor's tree hanged over his property, so he decided to get revenge by climbing the tree and cutting off the offending limb.

Probably would've been much easier situation to handle if the guy hadn't cut the limb while he was sitting on it.

Guy fell 20-something feet out of a tree, chainsaw's kill switch didn't activate properly for whatever reason, and the guy ended up almost chopping his own leg off in addition to injuries sustained in the fall.

This all happened after midnight, so we had to get spotlights out for EMS, and back at the station we all had to change our uniforms because we had blood all over us from trying to stabilize the patient until EMS arrived.

Guy wasn't even drunk.

-Y.N.
Virginia

Here's free medical advice: If you ever get the idea to hold a lit firecracker between your teeth, *don't.*

You don't even want to know all the injuries involved. I don't know how this patient is ever going to live a normal life again.

-Initials and location withheld at request

If you are going 35 MPH on a scooter and the 4,500-pound pickup truck that you're brake-checking out of road rage is going 55 MPH, it's not gonna end well if the driver hits you.

Patient did not die, but there were significant, critical injuries. Please, please, please buckle up your rage when you're out on the road. You never know what could happen!

-B.D.

Arizona

If it says on the package, "Not for human consumption," then that means DO NOT EAT IT.

The patient said of the laundry detergent pod, "I didn't eat it. I swallowed it like a pill."

Okay, well now you're admitted to ICU, so...

-P.F.

You should never set fireworks off indoors. If you *do* set fireworks off indoors, and said fireworks are the kind that shoot 50-feet in the air before exploding, you should probably pick a building that doesn't have 10-foot ceilings.

Multiple injuries, building evacuated, fire department called, and I'm preeeeety sure the people lost the security deposit they paid when they rented the wedding hall.

-Anonymous

Georgia

Kerry, I heard you said you weren't great at math, but here's an equation I'm sure you can figure out.

Stolen motorized hoverboard + neighbor's trampoline x (meth + alcohol) – safety gear – common sense = PT transport, arrest, and huge ER bill.

-E.M.
North Carolina

Exact words from our easiest arrest of the night: "Um, I have meth in wallet, too. Should I give that to you with my license and registration?"

Sure!

The lady said, "I'm going to jail? Wow, okay. I didn't think that was gonna happen for being honest."

-C.T.
Location withheld at request

Our patient participated in something called a 'Bird Box Challenge,' where he/she blindfolded themselves prior to chopping vegetables in the kitchen.

This patient was transported to the nearest ER...not for chopping a finger off, but for tripping over a box that was on the floor and banging his/her head on a counter.

I didn't know this 'challenge' existed until that call. Luckily, it was the only call we responded to for the 'challenge.'

The patient's friends were laughing about the incident, but the patient, who received sutures, was not.

Your friendly EMS staff does not support this 'challenge.' Don't wear a blindfold in the kitchen.

-K.S.

Arkansas

Fuming

My partner and I responded to an injury complaint. It had been difficult for us to race across town because it had been snowing all day. The roads were impossible to see. Forget about lanes. Basically, we used parked cars, trees, and our knowledge of the area to stay on what we thought were roads. Once we arrived on scene, we parked as close to the curb as we could, but I'm not sure how close that was because, like I said, there was just too much snow.

On scene, things weren't going so great. The patient had attempted to commit suicide by not only taking pills with alcohol, but additionally injuring him/herself in a manner that required immediate stabilization prior to transport.

We were in the patient's apartment approximately 15 to 20 minutes, give or take, before we could get the patient moved to the ambulance.

When we went outside, I was beyond shocked and disgusted. At the time, I'd been with EMS for five years or so, and I'd *never, ever* heard of this happening.

The city contracted a company to clear roadways during and following winter storms. This asshole, apparently, was angry because we parked in a 'No Parking' zone, so he had already plowed a mountain of snow in front of our ambulance, and he was in the process of blocking us in from behind as well. Our sirens were off, but our lights were still on! I mean, hello, if you can't tell that an ambulance with flashing lights parked on a street in the middle of the night isn't an emergency vehicle, then maybe you need to go back to school.

My partner ran out and stood between the plow and the back of our ambulance, but the guy in the plow didn't give two craps. My partner had to jump out of the way to avoid being packed in the wall of snow that the guy pushed right up against our vehicle.

Oh, I was so mad! Our patient needed to get to the ER ASAP. Waving our arms at the guy in the snow plow did nothing. He couldn't hear us screaming over the sound of his machine. I think he saw our patient on the stretcher, but I really don't think he cared. I don't know how he could look over and see the patient's crying family members and be proud of his behavior.

We notified dispatch of the problem. She contacted the police department. Nobody from the city could be contacted for this matter since it happened in the middle of the night, so we knew we weren't going to see immediate results.

The patient's family, the patient's neighbors, my partner, and I had to shovel the snow out of the way so we could load the patient and transport him/her to the ER. We worked as quickly as we could, but I think it still took about 10 minutes to get the back cleared and the patient loaded. It was total chaos.

Thankfully, the patient did not expire during transport (though it was close). The patient was admitted to Critical Care and received the help he/she needed in the weeks following the suicide attempt. Our supervisor, my partner, and I contacted the Streets and

Sanitation Department at the mayor's office, but we were met by the receptionist with, "Well, it's a no-parking zone. You shouldn't have been parked there."

We had to go over her head to file a formal complaint. From what I understand, the receptionist said she 'misunderstood' our complaint. We heard that the driver of the plow was suspended for three days. I don't wish bad against anyone, but I still am not sure that I agree with such a light punishment. Our patient could have *died* because this guy was so angry with our parking spot that he decided to behave vindictively and block us in.

I think the same driver managed the route by our station a while later, because one day both our lot exits were blocked off by huge mountains of hard snow. The station manager called for the situation to be remedied, but he was told by the plow company that they 'ran a tight schedule' and wouldn't be available to clear our exits for a few more hours. Our manager then hired a private individual to clear the exits, filed a complaint, and sent the plow bill to the city's contracted company. I think we caused so much of a stink over that, that it had to be noticed, because the following year the city had contracted out a different company.

I suppose it is what it is, now that it's been years later. We never encountered that issue again, but probably partially because when we park following a snow storm, we put cones around our vehicle, leave the lights on, and usually put a note on the driver's window that reads, "EMERGENCY RUN, DO NOT BLOCK VEHICLE."

-Anonymous
Colorado

Soda Pop

When I entered Jane and Joan's room to administer medication, Jane asked me, "Where's John? It's Wednesday, and he always gives us our pills on Wednesday. Is he sick?"

I probably should have kept my mouth shut, but I was upset that I had to work on a day I had scheduled off.

I sighed and spouted off in an irritated tone, "No, John is in jail because he was selling coke."

Jane looked confused and asked, "Since when did it become against the law to sell soda pop? What is this world coming to?"

I couldn't tell if she was serious, but I was pretty sure she was because she asked so innocently.

Joan looked over and said, "Honey, I think she meant John was dealing cocaine."

Jane laughed and said, "Oh. Well, maybe he should be in jail, then. We don't want that mess falling in the hands of children, right?"

I couldn't help but to laugh. It made my shift easier.

-C.D.

Kansas

Playing Around

For Christmas, my amazing wife purchased me an expensive interactive gaming system that included a firearm targeting practice scenario. With this kit, you load an electronic bullet in your personal firearm, which relays a signal to the gaming device. It's a pretty neat setup. I should add that I am an officer, but I had taken three weeks of PTO (Christmas miracle that will never occur again in my lifetime) and I had never left my house in uniform during that time.

I was testing out the system, when all the sudden our living room was lit up in flashing lights. There was a pounding at the door, so I put my firearm on the mantle of our fireplace, opened the door, and was met by a bunch of concerned armed officers. Six units had responded.

My new neighbor (whom my wife and I had not even met yet) called 911 because she saw through my open curtains that I was in the house, pointing a firearm. She thought my wife and children (my kids weren't home at the time of the incident—they were at grandma's house, thankfully) were in danger.

These officers worked with me daily, and we had gone through some rough calls together. We trusted each other fully, but they were still required to arrive on scene in a professional, guarded manner. They wanted to speak with my wife to make sure she felt safe. Then, as soon as they realized the call was a false alarm, they stuck around to check out my new system.

I send this to you because even though we work with men and women whom we can trust with our lives, you just never know what's going to happen at home. I also am sending you this because it's important to get to know your neighbors.

My wife and I introduced ourselves to our new neighbor the next day and explained my job and the gaming system. She apologized, but I told her there was no need to apologize. Had I moved into a new neighborhood and witnessed what she had, I also would have called in a complaint. I assured her that I am

a responsible firearm operator, in and out of
the house, and if she ever needed assistance,
she could call me day or night.

-J.W.

Kentucky

Intruder Alert

Dispatch received a 911 call at 02:30 from a neighbor regarding a noise complaint. The neighbor believed someone was breaking into the apartment next door, and she was especially concerned because the occupants were out of town for a funeral and weren't set to return until the following day.

We entered the apartment to find three cats had knocked down the occupants' Christmas tree. The tree smashed through a glass-top coffee table, and somehow, a mounted television had been knocked off the wall.

The place was a disaster. There were broken bulbs all over, glass from the table everywhere, and shiny garland had been dragged all over the apartment by these cats who all just froze when my partner and I walked inside. I don't speak cat, but I'm sure they were all telepathically saying to one another, "Oh crap, who's that? Should we move? Should we run off? Maybe if we stand real still, they won't think we did this."

Luckily, the neighbor had contact information for the occupants, so she called them. She also took the cats over to her apartment to prevent them from injuring themselves on the broken glass.

I went home that night and as I climbed in bed, my wife rolled over and said, "I think we should get [our daughter] a kitten."

I think my exact words were, "Hell no. I'll tame a moose before we get a cat."

We adopted an adult dog instead. The first thing he did when we brought him home was run wild through the house and knock over our Christmas tree.

I just can't win.

-N.T.
Pennsylvania

<u>Oh, Rats!</u>

I had recently moved into an apartment complex that wasn't in the best shape on the outside, but inside it didn't look so bad. I quickly learned that while you can slap a fresh coat of paint on old walls, you can't exactly hide old, shoddy plumbing or pest infestations.

On my first night in the apartment, I realized I had a roach infestation. Google told me that you can have roaches even if your residence is spotless, which is something I never knew. I hate bugs and called my landlord at 9 p.m. He didn't seem all that concerned, but he said he'd 'get someone out eventually.' I told him that for $1,700 a month, he'd better get someone out *tomorrow.* He hung up on me.

An exterminator came in while I was at work (with my permission), but he left a note that said he couldn't spray any chemicals or put down traps because he noticed my cat was roaming around the living room. I contacted his business and scheduled him to come the next day. I made plans to take my cat to a friend's house and let him stay the night there or stay there until it was safe for him to come home.

The stress of moving made me tired, but the idea of bugs crawling around my apartment kept me awake. I finally fell asleep around 01:00. I had to be up for work at 04:30. I told myself that if I skipped a shower and styling my hair, I could sleep until 05:00.

I heard my cat making all kinds of noise, so I woke up, saw that it was 03:00, and I told him to go to bed. I then fell back asleep.

A few minutes later, I felt something heavy on my chest, and I can't even describe the smell. Ugh.

I opened my eyes to find my cat gripping a RAT that he'd set on my chest. The thing was still alive. It was so huge that I have no freaking idea how my cat even managed to pick it up. I don't think he could have killed it even if he wanted to. He had apparently just been dragging it around the apartment and decided, 'Hey, I wonder if my mom's ever seen one of these?'

When I screamed, my cat let go of the rodent, which then ran over my face and behind my bed. My cat followed the same path, chased the rat under the bed, and then I watched the rat and my cat bolt across the bedroom and into the bathroom. I ran to the kitchen for a broom, only to see roaches scatter all over when I turned on the light, and then I ran back to the bathroom, only to watch this rat disappear down the pipe in my toilet. I freaked out when I saw it wriggle its way out of the toilet. As this soaking wet monstrosity came at me, I tripped over my cat, hit my head on the sink (and broke the sink off the wall in the process), and then I somehow managed to stab myself in the eye with the broom handle.

I had to call 911 because I was bleeding so much from my head that I thought I was dying. The ER doctor said I had hit it in 'just the right spot,' but it wasn't anything to be concerned about. He said I scratched my eye up pretty good, so he prescribed me drops and told me to wear a patch for a while. I called off from work and looked like a sleep-deprived pirate when I went to my landlord's office the next morning. My landlord just kind of shrugged it off.

My saving grace in all this was the exterminator found a major mold problem when he arrived, so I was able to get out of my lease. The landlord didn't want to return my deposit or my rent (citing a contract and the damage to the sink), so I had to stay with my friend until I could get my finances figured out. I eventually had to threaten to take the landlord to court. He finally returned my money.

I now rent a small duplex and have not seen any pests/rodents yet. I think I've seen enough to last a lifetime.

-P.L.
Texas

O, Christmas Tree

I'm not sure what would possess our patient (well-dressed man in his 30s, driving a nice sports car, in for a complaint of sore throat) to steal the 4-ft Christmas tree from our waiting room, but I'm not sure he thought out his escape route.

Plastic bulbs were dropping in a tell-tale trail behind him, a strand of lights got caught on a chair and unraveled until the tree was naked, and then…THEN, the man tried to run through the door with the tree held horizontally in his arms.

You can't take a 4-ft tree through a 2-ft opening without turning it sideways or *something*.

The guy bounced back like he'd been electrocuted. He was lying on his back with the tree over his torso as security approached him.

A guard said, "That probably wasn't the smartest thing you've ever done, huh?"

The patient said, "No, I don't think so."

Security walked the patient to his vehicle and told him not to come back unless he needed medical assistance.

I dragged the tree back to the waiting room and kind of threw the lights and bulbs back on it. The poor thing looked so pitiful. The top of the tree was bent from where it got caught on the door frame, so it looked like the tree was hanging its head in embarrassment. I really don't know why he wanted our tree in the first place because I think they seriously bought it back in 1987. The thing smells disgusting, like dust and mold. It's ugly as sin, with faded needles and bald patches.

I was clicking through our local news website a few days later and saw the patient's mugshot listed. He had been arrested for theft on the same day he tried to steal our tree.

-W.A.
Oregon

Sounded Like a Good Idea at the Time

Our 30-something-year-old patient said he saw a video on Facebook of a pocket rocket that had a curved loop over the top. The driver was able to tilt the cycle forward, drive upside down on the curved loop device, and then drive upright again.

Thinking this would be an awesome thing to be able to do himself, the patient fixed a thin slat of wood over his cycle and attempted to drive upside down…while driving 50+ MPH.

The friend who was filming called 911 because the wood snapped in half. The patient fell off the cycle, landed on his head, and the cycle went catapulting forward, where it crashed into the side of the patient's father's truck.

This story was consistent with the fact that two officers were holding the patient's father at a distance, trying to convince him to drop his leather belt…which he'd used to beat the patient while everyone was waiting for help to arrive.

The patient sustained multiple contusions and lacerations from the wreck. He also suffered from a sprained neck. He complained of soreness in the locations where his father beat him with the belt. When the patient told us (EMS) that he wanted to press charges, the father exploded, "Press charges? You live here rent-free and do nothing but sit around and play on your phone!" The officers moved the father inside in an attempt keep the scene calm.

I don't know what happened after that, but I would estimate the damage to the truck to be at least $1,500, and the cycle was basically totaled.

-J.S.
North Carolina

Should've Listened

I was walking to work one day, when I passed by a couple arguing on a staircase that led to a second-story apartment.

The woman said to a man, "Do you want a broken leg? Because that's how you get a broken leg."

He replied, "Jane, why do you have to ruin everything?"

She shouted, "Because you just tried to rollerblade down the stairs! But if you really have your heart set on spending the afternoon in the emergency room, don't let me stop you."

I heard him say, "No, you're right. I won't do it."

An hour later, I was the responding medic to that residence. The man had gone along with his plan…and it was clear he'd broken his leg. I never followed up with the ER, but I'm pretty sure his wrist was messed up, too.

I guess the woman wasn't home because the man said, "Man, my girlfriend is gonna be so pissed when she finds out I actually did it."

I don't think he recognized me as a passerby, and I didn't know if it would be appropriate to tell him that I'd heard the conversation from earlier, so I just kept my mouth shut.

-T.G.

California

Negative Reviews

We responded to a complaint of a loud, violent customer at our small-town movie theater. There was Jane, our local critic. She prided herself on leaving reviews for **ev-er-y-thing**, so if our coffee shop created a Facebook page, you can bet Jane would be the first one on there to leave a review.

There's really nothing wrong with leaving reviews, but Jane could never leave a *positive* review.

There's also nothing wrong with that, but she'd find stupid reasons to leave bad reviews.

For example, Jane left a review for the coffee shop that read, "Coffee was way too hot. I had to let it cool down for five minutes before I could even drink it. You guys need to learn how to make coffee."

She left another review a few weeks later that read, "The caramel iced coffee I ordered was too cold, and the caramel didn't taste like the kind I buy in stores. Avoid at all costs."

She seemed to think that her opinion was God, and if anyone thought otherwise, she would get herself in some mighty trouble.

That was the case when we arrived at the theater. Jane had demanded a refund for the movie she'd just watched. The theater's owner, however, refused to issue a refund. When he refused, Jane screamed and screamed. Her temper worsened, until she finally ripped the cash register off the counter and then kicked a hole in the glass counter. Nobody wanted to get too close to her because she was acting like a monster.

We placed Jane under arrest because she couldn't control her temper and she refused to comply with our orders. The last straw was when she spit on one of my deputies.

"They need to give me my money back," Jane screamed. "That movie was fake. That could never, ever happen. It wasn't real at all."

"Of course it wasn't, you psycho," the owner of the theater shouted. "You just watched Harry [effing] Potter!"

The owner went on to explain that if the theater had been at fault for Jane's disappointment, he would have gladly issued a refund. However, the theater had not had issues regarding volume, playback, snacks, cleanliness, safety, or comfort of seating, so the owner refused to issue a refund just because Jane didn't like the movie.

I stopped what I was doing and asked the theater owner, "Harry Potter? You're showing Harry Potter?"

He nodded and told me it was part of a promotional summer showing for kids. I thought the movie was okay and wouldn't mind seeing it in theater again, so I shrugged and told him I'd be back later.

Jane assured us that she would leave a review to let everyone know what kind of jail our county 'really' had. I think the internet gave her some kind of inflated ego that made her think that she was going to lead the revolution on county jails or something, I don't know.

Jane's family refused to bail her out (shocker), so we had the great pleasure of having her in our facility for five days before she had her court date. She was ordered to make payments to the movie theater to repair the counter and register, and she was given probation.

She went right back to leaving her reviews, but we haven't had a (major) problem with her since then.

-Initials and location withheld at request

The Little Things

We had a teenager come in right after school to ask us if we could cut his hair and write a note to tell his mom that it was medically necessary. He said he couldn't pay us anything, but he volunteered to clean in exchange for our services.

When I tell this story to my friends and new RNs, they always ask, "Why? Was his hair really long or something?"

His mother cut his hair because it saved the family money, and the only haircut she knew how to do was a bowl cut. The kid was about 14 or 15-years-old and had never had a 'modern' hairstyle. He was so upset when we told him no that he started crying and telling us that everyone bullied him for his hair, and that he couldn't just cut it off because his mom would be upset. He showed us bruises on his back from where he stated classmates punched him when they teased him. It was really sad, but we couldn't really do anything.

I slipped the kid $20 and told him how to find the barber where I take my sons. He came back to show me his brand-new haircut, and he cried as he thanked me.

The very next day, the kid came back with his mother. I thought she was going to scream at me. She thanked me. She was a single mother to three kids, and she worked three jobs. She was in tears when she told me that she didn't know her son had been bullied until he came home with his new haircut. She started saving $20 every other month so her son could continue to get his hair cut by a professional, and her son would come in every few months to show me a new style.

I never even treated the kid as a patient, but that was one of my proudest and most rewarding moments in nursing.

-J.C.
New York

If you're going to fly a paramotor (like a go-kart-type vehicle with a parachute fixed to the top that allows you to fly through the air), then you should make sure you're buckled in and wearing proper safety gear.

Our patient broke 10+ bones because the vehicle turned while 20+ feet off the ground. No idea how the patient lived. Lucky, I guess.

-F.G.

Ohio

Beware of Cat

Our elderly patient told dispatch to tell us, "Watch out for the cat."

We thought the patient meant, "Don't let the cat out when you come in for this lift assist."

When we entered the house and made sure we didn't let the cat out, we thought we were all good. As soon as my partner walked around the corner, this 20-something-pound cat leapt out of the darkness, covered my partner's face with its body, clung to him by digging its claws in his neck, and bit at my partners face and ears.

My partner was so beat up that our supervisor sent him to the ED for a checkup. It was crazy.

-L.B.
Louisiana

Our patient's husband was bored and couldn't sit still. He picked up an instrument from the table at the patient's bedside, held it up in the air, and asked, "What is this, like an antenna or something?"

He opened his mouth and pretended to pick his teeth. He said, "It's a fancy toothpick, isn't it?"

"Sir," I scolded, "please put that down. It's a uterine sound."

"What's that mean?" he asked, still waving the device around and placing it centimeters from his face.

"That's used to dilate the uterus," I said.

He dropped the instrument immediately and ran to the bathroom.

-M.L.
Mississippi

I came out of the bathroom to see a patient standing in the lobby, staring down his reflection in the two-way security mirror.

The patient then began arguing with his reflection and shouted, "Get out of my [effing] way, man!"

He punched the 'unbreakable' mirror and cracked it.

"Sir!" I shouted, "You're arguing with your reflection!"

He showed me his bleeding fist, puked on the floor, and then passed out.

I'm not sure why he came to ES in the first place, but he was so drunk that they kept him overnight for observation.

-T.F.
New Jersey

<u>Getting Out of a Ticket</u>

I pulled over a middle-aged man for speeding. I can't even remember how fast he was going, maybe 15 or 20 over the posted limit.

While I was standing at his door, trying to ask for his license, I kept getting distracted. I couldn't even form a full sentence without trailing off.

Finally, I broke down and asked him, "Sir, it's probably none of my business, but why do you have a sex toy suctioned to your dashboard?"

He shrugged and said, "I don't know. I bought it for my wife, but she didn't want to use it. Can't take it back to the store, so might as well use it for something. I thought it'd be funny to put there."

I didn't give him a ticket because I couldn't conduct myself in a professional manner. I told him to slow it down, and then I went back to my cruiser to giggle like a 13-

year-old boy after seeing the hot pink 12-inch silicone penis flopping every which way.

-R.R.
Oklahoma

<u>Distracted Driving</u>

I was parked in a lot that faced a busy roadway, hoping that my presence would slow some drivers down and deter them from making illegal decisions. Especially during rush hour, that road is known for wrecks and traffic jams.

I noticed there was a holdup at the roundabout down the way. Traffic was backed up. Everyone was honking. There was this one sedan, just parked at a stop sign, holding up traffic.

I moved my vehicle closer, parked and exited, and then walked over to the vehicle. I became furious when I saw the driver was holding up traffic because he was watching a video on his phone. I tapped on the glass.

He looked up at me, surprised and fearful. He slowly lowered his window.

"Seriously?" I asked. "You're *seriously* holding everyone up, just so you can play with your phone? I know you could see my car over there. You thought it was a good idea to hold up traffic with an officer nearby, just so you could play on your phone?"

The fear of God was in this man, and I thought he was going to cry.

He turned the screen for me to see and he admitted, "Nobody was behind me when I stopped. I don't know how to do this."

He was watching a YouTube video that explained how to use a roundabout.

I didn't know what to say, so I just kind of chuckled and asked, "Well, do you think you understood the video enough to move out of the way?"

He nodded and asked if I was going to write him a ticket.

I should have, but I think I was so floored by what he had been doing that my brain wouldn't allow it.

-M.W.
Indiana

A Message to Readers

If you follow me on social media, you'll probably recognize some of the following as being shared earlier. I wanted to share it again for readers who don't follow me online, just because I like to connect with all my readers.

Following my last two books, I received some feedback and wanted to clarify a few things with everyone.

Stories included in the 'Reader Submission' series come from readers like you. I do my best to edit submissions in a way that tell the readers' stories without taking out too much of their personalities. Please know that I would never knowingly disparagingly describe a person's disability, illness, or addiction. I know I use a lot of sarcasm and humor in these books, but I'm very serious when it comes to treating others with respect, and despite the snarky things I've spoken and/or thought in humorous hindsight, I'd never dream of treating someone poorly or offensively. One submission used the term 'handicapable,' which is a term some find offensive. I completely understand why some take offense to it. This term was used by the reader who submitted the story, and I did not feel comfortable changing the reader's words (nor did I ask if I could change the words). There's a difference in making light of something a person does or says versus a person's condition, and I won't do the latter because I think that's cruel, not funny.

The submissions that I include do not necessarily reflect my personal beliefs. You will see that I often include an author's note if I have anything to add. I added an author's note on a story about a pit bull attack, and I may not have clarified my opinion on the topic. It wasn't my intention to 'preach' or 'rant' about my opinions, and my opinions weren't breed-specific. I simply meant that I believe some dogs are predisposed to display certain tendencies, but ANY dog can react in any manner. Sorry for the miscommunication there. I've received a few messages and think I should note that I don't have anything against pit bulls or pit mixes; *I own one.* He's almost 55-pounds, loves cats and kids, enjoys car rides and trips to the store to pick his own toys, and he's the gentlest dog I know (but knows when to be a guard dog/crime deterrent). Definitely don't have anything against the breed. I also own a 14-year-old 15-pound dog who's a demon spawn, and I have an 11-year-old 80-pound dog who's old and just wants everyone to leave her alone and let her sleep half the time. Trust me, I'm an advocate for all dog breeds to be treated fairly!

Some people have expressed frustration with the length of my books, specifically the mini I last released. While most of the feedback was lighthearted (and appreciated), some of it was…Well, let's just say I received some nasty messages. I think it's easy to disconnect from people we see or hear from in any form of media. As I've stated before, I'm neither rich nor famous. I'm an ordinary person (well, I'm pretty weird and introverted, but you get the idea) with a house full of pets, bills to pay, a personal life (not much of one, but enough of one), and problems like everyone else. I do freelance work throughout the week and write to fill the rest of the time. I also write for children and write other adult content, so just because you don't see a hospital book doesn't mean I'm not working on something.

Now that all that's out of the way, let's go to the usual stuff. Thank you for all your support! Thanks for all the comments and Twitter tags! I enjoy keeping in touch with everyone, and I'm grateful to have you all around on social media. You guys sure know how to keep it fun. I'm hoping not to have any backlash over the 'Funny Florida' section, but I suppose time will tell, right?

I've finished just in time for a snowstorm, so I'm sure you'll see me complaining about that on social media soon enough.

Try to stay warm, stay same, and have a great day!

Check me out on Twitter!

https://twitter.com/AuthorKerryHamm

You can also find me on Facebook, by searching for 'Author Kerry Hamm.'

www.ingramcontent.com/pod-product-compliance
Lightning Source LLC
Chambersburg PA
CBHW030610220526
45463CB00004B/1238